One Body, One Life

Gregory Joujon-Roche

and

CAMERON STAUTH

DUTTON

One Body,

6 *Weeks* *to the*

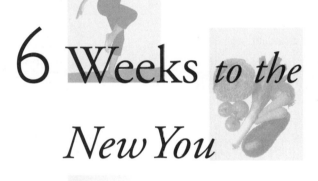

New You

One **Life**

Every effort has been made to ensure that the information contained in this book is complete and accurate. However, neither the author nor the publisher is engaged in rendering professional advice or services to the individual reader. The ideas, procedures, and suggestions contained in this book are not intended as a substitute for consulting your physician. All matters regarding your health require medical supervision. Neither the author not the publisher shall be liable or responsible for any loss, injury, or damage allegedly arising from any information or suggestions in this book.

DUTTON
Published by Penguin Group (USA) Inc.
375 Hudson Street, New York, New York 10014, U.S.A.
Penguin Group (Canada), 90 Eglinton Avenue East, Suite 700, Toronto, Ontario M4P 2Y3, Canada (a division of Pearson Penguin Canada Inc.); Penguin Books Ltd, 80 Strand, London WC2R 0RL, England; Penguin Ireland, 25 St Stephen's Green, Dublin 2, Ireland (a division of Penguin Books Ltd); Penguin Group (Australia), 250 Camberwell Road, Camberwell, Victoria 3124, Australia (a division of Pearson Australia Group Pty Ltd); Penguin Books India Pvt Ltd, 11 Community Centre, Panchsheel Park, New Delhi - 110 017, India; Penguin Group (NZ), cnr Airborne and Rosedale Roads, Albany, Auckland 1310, New Zealand (a division of Pearson New Zealand Ltd); Penguin Books (South Africa) (Pty) Ltd, 24 Sturdee Avenue, Rosebank, Johannesburg 2196, South Africa

Penguin Books Ltd, Registered Offices: 80 Strand, London WC2R 0RL, England

Published by Dutton, a member of Penguin Group (USA) Inc.

First printing, April 2006
10 9 8 7 6 5 4 3 2 1

REGISTERED TRADEMARK—MARCA REGISTRADA

LIBRARY OF CONGRESS CATALOGING-IN-PUBLICATION DATA
Joujon-Roche, Gregory.
    One body, one life : 6 weeks to the new you / by Gregory Joujon-
Roche and Cameron Stauth.
        p.   cm.
    ISBN 0-525-94919-4 (hardcover)
    1. Physical fitness.   2. Exercise   I. Stauth, Cameron.   II. Title.
Title: One body, one life : six weeks to the new you.
GV481.J696 2006
613.7'1—dc22

Printed in the United States of America
Set in Adobe Garamond
Designed by Kate Nichols

While the author has made every effort to provide accurate telephone numbers and Internet addresses at the time of publication, neither the publisher nor the author assumes any responsibility for errors, or for changes that occur after publication. Further, publisher does not have any control over and does not assume any responsibility for author or third-party Web sites or their content.

For Irma and Dylan

Contents

Acknowledgments

The authors would like to gratefully acknowledge the important contributions to this book that were provided by our accomplished colleagues.

Brian Tart, president and publisher of Dutton, believed that the genre of fitness books could be elevated to a higher, more meaningful level, and he worked hard to make this belief a reality.

Neil Gordon edited this book with tremendous energy, creativity, and intelligence, guiding everything from the big picture to the smallest detail. His influence is on every page.

Richard Pine, of InkWell Management—the true man behind the scenes: thank you for believing.

Matthew Guma, of InkWell Management, made this book happen. His vision is changing the face of fitness.

Sharon House and I met four years ago, and none of this would have been possible without her. Sharon, you're always there.

Yumi Lee, Tanja Djelevic, and Steven Ho—the heart and soul of Holistic Fitness—provided the Workout expertise that has put them among the leading fitness experts of our era.

Thanks to my whole team at Holistic Fitness: Stephen Jochen, Stephanie and Stephen Koff, Stephen Barton, Paul McReynolds, Sara Ivanhoe, John Platero, Greg and Dianne Isaacs, Diviana Ingravalo, Daneen Flesher, Nathan Allen, and Gee Linton.

Irma, my wife, also offered inestimable help in the areas of yoga and nutrition—and everything, it seems. Thank you, my true love.

Sandra Stahl, working on her eleventh book, brought order and clarity to a process that is inescapably chaotic.

Kevin Huvane, director of Creative Artists Agency, turned hopes and dreams into action and accomplishment. He is the reason Holistic Fitness exists. He believed in me from the start, when I was training out of my apartment. The bad parking, bad area, and scary elevator rides made for a friendship that will last lifetimes.

My friends at Waterfront Media, especially Steven Petrow, ignited a spark of excitement and promise that kept us going. Steven, keep wearing the jeans.

Jose Pombo, the most rock 'n' roll angel of a photographer and human on the planet: Thanks!

Thanks to my mom, dad, and Nancy, and my Sista, for always being there.

And so many other people helped, from my clients to their assistants, publicists, and everybody in between.

This was a group effort in the biggest way. Thank you, everyone, for believing in me and supporting this grand venture.

—*Gregory Joujon-Roche*

My heartfelt thanks to the people who have helped the most: Brian, Neil, Richard, Matthew, and Sandra. You all know how appreciative I am.

—*Cameron Stauth*

One Body, One **Life**

Part

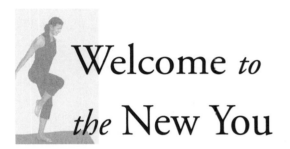

Welcome *to* *the* New You

One

Here's *You*—
Six Weeks from Now

Let's begin at the end. At the end of the next six weeks, how do you see yourself? Take a moment and visualize it.

Here's what I think you see: a slimmer and healthier you, with tighter muscles, a flatter stomach, a greater glow of energy, and a feeling of empowerment. I think you see an image of change.

If you did, good. Helping people change is my business, and my passion.

It's exciting for me to work with people who really want to change. My company, Holistic Fitness, works primarily with movie stars, rock stars, and high-octane executives—the kind of people who love change, and demand results.

Many other, less committed people, I'm certain, buy fitness books and join health clubs for a very different reason: to keep from feeling guilty. They just want to go through the motions, without breaking a sweat. It makes them feel good just to own a fitness book, or to belong to a gym.

These people do not really want to change. For them, it's just too much trouble.

What makes me think you're not one of them? Because I know you could have found a less realistic fitness book. There are all kinds of hokey books out there that say all you need to do is work out three times a week for ten minutes to look fabulous. You could have picked one of those.

But apparently you're too savvy for that. You know that change never comes from doing just ten minutes of work, three times a week. You know that reward comes from commitment. And you know that this commitment can be fun.

Most of all, you know this: You have only one body, and you have only one life—so it's smart to be serious about them.

This sounds like common sense, but you'd be amazed at how many people just don't get it.

Look around you. You see people treating their bodies so badly that they must think that someday they can get a "body transplant." You see people living their lives as if this life is just a practice session for the real thing.

If these people were to visualize themselves in six weeks' time, they would probably see the same-old same-old. No differences. No change.

They might, in fact, think that it's not even possible to achieve fundamental change in just six weeks.

They're wrong.

It's entirely possible to make dramatic changes in your body in six weeks. I frequently have even less than six weeks to help movie stars transform their bodies for specific roles. These roles are extraordinarily demanding: action hero, glamour symbol, and even comic book superhero. Try looking like that in six weeks.

The only possible way to achieve this degree of body transformation in such a short time is with an all-encompassing, full-scale program. The main reason my One Body, One Life program creates such fast and lasting results is because it is comprehensive yet accessible. It addresses all four of the most fundamental elements of fitness and health.

1. **Mind and Spirit:** The only masters of the body.
2. **Power Food:** The food that builds the body, without burdening it.
3. **Cleansing:** The procedures that get rid of energy-destroying toxins.
4. **Exercise:** The action that burns fat and builds muscle.

Each of the Four Elements of Fitness is addressed almost every day during your six-week program. Each reinforces the others. The combined synergistic power of all four is overwhelming.

Therefore, you will make progress every day on the One Body, One Life program. Each day, your body will become more toned, and you'll be slimmer. This transformation will make every successive day a little bit easier.

To ensure that you will keep making incremental progress, the program is divided into three phases.

Phase One: This is the two-week start-up stage, during which you do the easiest workouts, and learn the basics of good nutrition, internal cleansing, and using your mental power to change your body.

As in the following two phases, your Phase-One Workouts will be the epitome of cross-training in order to hit every muscle group and banish boredom. Monday is Strength Workout Day. Tuesday is Yoga Day. Wednesday is Pilates Day. Thursday is Martial Arts Day. Friday is Core Interval Training Day. Never a dull moment. And don't worry: no experience necessary. Just show up, and let me take care of the rest.

Phase Two: This is the two-week period in the middle of the program. At this stage, the five days of Workouts get turned up a notch, for even more results, and the information on food, cleansing, and the mind gets more detailed. Get ready for your first weekend cleanse, to make you feel light and bright.

Phase Three: This is the last two weeks, in which you transform yourself physically and mentally into the person you want to be. The Workouts are in full throttle, and the information on mind, food, and cleansing is very specific and sophisticated.

By the end of these three phases, believe me, you won't look the same. Or feel the same.

How can you really change in just six weeks? Simple: by engaging in a full-scale program that taps the power you already have. The human body has amazing potential. Think about it. If you follow the program for the next six weeks, you will lose weight, gain lean muscle, increase your vitality and endurance, and feel better about how you look. The beauty of the body is that it always responds to improvements in diet and exercise habits. Every effort you make will be rewarded.

Over these same six weeks, your mind and spirit will also undergo noticeable changes. You just can't do this work without adjusting your attitude. Your mind and body will have to be in sync. You'll learn to stop indulging in fear and negative expectations. You'll learn how to focus on your physical powers, and how to then go beyond focus, into the realm of exercise-as-meditation.

During the six weeks, you'll also begin to clear your body of toxins. Draining the poisons from your body will make you feel young again.

As you subtract fat and toxins, you'll add lean muscle, and jump-start your metabolism. You will become more toned, lithe, and firm. Every part of your body will improve, from your butt to your biceps. And you'll see great improvement in your core—especially your abdominal area.

In addition, you will also experience tremendous improvement over the next six weeks in things that you can't see, but can feel—such as your energy level, your mood, your cognitive ability, and even your ability to sleep well. These changes will feel so great that they'll become virtually addictive.

The reason all this will happen in just six weeks is because of the synergistic details of the program. The fine-tuning that I've been doing over the past ten years has really paid off. I've learned which specific exercises help the most, and exactly how to perform them.

Over the past decade, I've been teaching my One Body, One Life program everywhere from India to London, and Los Angeles to Australia. I have trained a sultan, a knight, a prince, rock stars, movie stars, athletes—and everyone in between. I'll share all this with you. In just six weeks, you'll learn:

- How staying full can make you slim.
- How food reactions can make you fat.
- How to be slim for the rest of your life without dieting.
- Why spot reducing is a media myth.
- How to find time to exercise, even when you have no time.

And that's just the beginning.

All of this information is packaged in this book in very short pieces that are easy to read. As you can see, a lot of this book looks more like a fun, reader-friendly magazine than a boring book on fitness. That's because serious information doesn't have to be boring, or exhausting.

There's never been a book like this.

There's never been a program like this.

If you stick with it, you will succeed.

Chapter 2

The Star Treatment

Here's Demi Moore, trying to do the impossible: a set of one-armed push-ups—done properly, with her hand almost under her chin, instead of splayed way out in front—and it hurts just to watch.

We're on the movie set of *G.I. Jane* and Demi's tightrope-taut muscles are shivering like Jell-O, but if any of these crew members standing around think she's going to give up, it's because they don't know her like I do. The reason she's so capable of projecting strength in her movie roles is because she's got it: You can't project what you don't have, even in the movies. Especially in the movies, to be honest about it. The big screen is brutally revealing. Lesser actors can fake their way through little roles, but virtually all the blue-chip superstars look bigger than life onscreen for a very simple reason: They really are bigger than life. They are willing to do things, and to experience things, that would humble the average actor.

There are thousands of actors who want to have what superstars have, but hardly any of them want to do what superstars do.

Such as: a set of one-armed push-ups. They're hard enough for an athletic male to do. When Sly Stallone did some in *Rocky*, it was a big deal, and got used in many of the movie's publicity stills. But women just don't have the anatomical composition of fast-twitch muscles that make repeated one-armed push-ups possible.

Demi, though, loves the fact that it's next to impossible. She's got no fear—doesn't understand the meaning of the word, as the expression goes.

Even so, one-armed push-ups are so hard that the stunt coordinator goes off and rigs up this spring-loaded device that my client can wear over her arm, to give her a little help. She takes one look at it and says, in so many words, no thank you.

Then we spend weeks building her up, doing extremely specific exercises to ignite the exact muscle groups she'll need. At the same time, we're doing all this Navy SEAL–style training, which is the polar opposite of prior work she'd done with me for glamour-type roles, such as her starring role in *Striptease*. In the glamour roles, we'd trained her for sexy and svelte, with dancing, aerobics, and gymnastics. But now she needs a completely different type of body—an action-hero body—so we're locked into this torturous boot-camp regimen of sit-ups in the mud, jumping jacks in quicksand, jogging underwater—that sort of thing. "Cold? Too bad! Get back in the water!" as the SEALs would say.

Demi is very patient about all this, but the truth is, she's been around the block with personal trainers and all of their demands. Most of what they've told her, she's already heard, and most of what they know about, she knows more. She is as savvy about her own body as anyone in Hollywood. You don't become a superstar by accident. So if somebody like me says, "Get back in the water!" I'd better have a very specific outcome in mind, and a very finite timetable.

Most people think that stars have all the time in the world to make themselves look good. They just go to expensive spas and get the star treatment, right? I can't count the number of times that the nonactor clients I train have said, "I'd look great, too, if that was my whole job." Well, fitness isn't an actor's whole job. Believe me, a superstar's life is ridiculously time consuming, from preproduction to press appearances. Likely as not, when a superstar arrives at my gym, his or her assistant will say, "We've got thirty minutes." And if I start to complain, he'll say, "We've now got twenty-nine and a half."

Time counts. For everybody. Including you, no doubt. That's part of the reason my approach is now so popular in Hollywood—it achieves maximum results in minimal time.

Another reason this one-armed push-up is such a challenge is because of the unavoidable pressure that always comes from studios, directors, and producers. They invariably have hundreds of millions of dollars riding on my ability to get a star into the exact shape the role requires. Do you think they want to hear excuses? Do they want to deal with injuries? Exercise burnout? Exhaustion? Weight that won't be gone for another ten days?

They want one thing: results. Now. Or, preferably, yesterday. That's why my approach is so specific, detailed, and outcome-oriented. The movie business is the wrong place for fuzzy philosophies and fake, feel-good exercise formulas.

Because directors live and die by their shooting schedules, timing is everything to them, and now it's time: time for Demi to do an unassisted, one-armed push-up.

I get down on the floor with her. I'm sweating, too—just from empathy. That often happens when I direct a workout, because I'm so wired in to the client that I feel like it's happening to me, too. Their pain is my pain.

I start breaking down the mechanics of a one-armed push-up in minute detail. Fitness is all about detail. **If you're not doing it right, you're not doing it.** You will see this line again and again throughout the book.

"A one-armed push-up doesn't come from your shoulder," I tell her. "It comes from your butt. From your stomach. Most especially, it comes from the big toe on the opposite side of your supporting arm. It's all about distributing your power. It's a support-system move, even more than a power move."

I see the proverbial lightbulb click on in her head. This explanation is all it takes for her to get it.

She gets into position. Painfully lowers her nose to the floor. Fights to rise back up. Her tricep is twitching.

She's hit the Breakthrough Moment, the do-or-die moment of muscle memory in which all fitness occurs—or doesn't, if you back off.

In that moment, as often happens in the Breakthrough Moment, I can see her own personal relationship with herself. It's right there on her face. It's very complex, and very positive.

She's up!

She grins at me. "That was good," she says, wiping her face with a snow-white towel.

"That was great!" I reply. "Yumi taught me that," I say, referring to Yumi Lee, my specialist in core interval training.

Yumi is one of several people in my personal training firm who makes us the best in the world at what we do. I'm smart enough to surround myself with people who are smarter than I.

We shoot the scene, and it ends up being one of the most remembered sequences in the movie. It gets featured in a bunch of magazines, and Demi goes on Letterman and does some there.

Here's what I learned from all this: Even the impossible can be achieved, if you use the right approach. You've just got to know exactly what you're doing.

You have to be smart about it. And that starts with breaking your beliefs in the myths that surround fitness.

BUSTING THE SIX BIG FITNESS MYTHS

- Fitness doesn't come from suffering.
- Fitness doesn't come from repetitive exercises.
- Fitness doesn't come from lifting oversized weights.
- Fitness doesn't come from being hungry.
- Fitness doesn't come from being dissatisfied with how you look.
- Fitness doesn't come from putting your appearance first.

You know, I almost wish all these myths were true. Life would be simpler. Because it's not that hard to do repetitive exercises. It's not that hard to be hungry. It's not even that hard to suffer. You just need some discipline to do those things, and almost all of us have discipline. The vast majority of us make ourselves go to work every day, whether we feel like it or not. All our lives, we hold ourselves back from the temptations of overindulgence, promiscuity, and drugs. We take care of our kids, day after day, when we're sick and when we're well. Most of us are strong—plenty strong enough to be fit.

The real problem, for most people, is that they just don't know how to be fit.

I know how, though.

I've made it my life's work to know how. I've been fascinated by fitness ever since I was a kid, and I've worked on it ever since. I've figured out the formula.

FITNESS REQUIRES: A COORDINATED EFFORT ON EVERY LEVEL OF YOUR LIFE.

- The Physical Level
- The Mental Level
- The Spiritual Level

If you try to leave one level out, you'll end up feeling like a three-legged stool with one leg missing. You'll fall. You'll fail.

And let's get even more honest with ourselves—painfully honest. To get all three of these areas working together—as a single, synchronistic, functional unit—you've got to participate in a multifaceted program that addresses all three.

I have developed a program that does this. I call this program my One Body, One Life program. It is a multifaceted program that brings your body and your life together, into a single, powerful life force.

When your whole being is united, there is practically nothing that you cannot do.

Unity is power. With it, you can achieve the hard things in life, including fitness, naturally—without much strain, and without fighting yourself—because you will be. . . .

How do I say this without sounding all New Age and woo-woo?

. . . Aligned with the forces of the universe? (No, too woo-woo.)

. . . In touch with the natural rhythms of the earth? (Oh, please!)

. . . At peace with yourself? (That's closer.)

How about this? You'll be somebody who has more energy. That's what it boils down to.

When you get yourself together, instead of staying compartmentalized—with your mind at work, your body in the gym, and your spirit at church—you'll have more energy.

And when you have more energy, you'll use it. Because it's harder to sit on energy than it is to burn it off.

When you use it, you'll get fit.

My One Body, One Life program consists of four connected elements: the Four Elements of Fitness.

THE FOUR ELEMENTS OF FITNESS

Element #1: Mind and Spirit: getting your head right.
Element #2: Power Food: eating for your body, not against it.
Element #3: Cleansing: cleaning out the toxins that weigh you down.
Element #4: Exercise: getting the most out of the body you've got.

These Four Elements of Fitness will give you power over the one body that you have, and power over the one life that you have.

If you use these Four Elements of Fitness on a daily basis, nothing will stop you from getting the body, and the life, that you want.

If you can integrate these four simple elements into your life, as so many other people have, you will be a star—playing the lead role in the story of your life.

> **A Gentle Reminder . . .**
>
> This book is not about *movie stars*. It's about YOU.
>
> (And how you can be the star of your own life.)

What's Your Fitness IQ?

ROUND ONE

Answer "true" or "false" for each question.

1. For weight management, it doesn't matter when you eat—all that really matters is how much. **T F**

2. You lose more weight from moderate exercise, during which you can still carry on a conversation, than you do from strenuous exercise, when you're breathing too hard to talk. **T F**

3. Weight work builds muscles, but isn't nearly as effective for weight loss as aerobics. **T F**

4. It's a fact of life: As you age, your metabolism slows significantly and causes extra weight gain. **T F**

5. Men and women face essentially the same challenges in becoming fit. To presume that women have a naturally harder time is an example of a self-defeating attitude. **T F**

6. Nonstrenuous movement during the day has little impact on fitness and weight management. People need to face the fact that hard work is all that really helps. **T F**

7. One of the more difficult challenges of fitness is that the more you exercise, the more you want to eat. **T F**

8. It's normal, and even desirable, to feel depleted and tired after exercise. It's the single most reliable sign that you did a sufficient amount. **T F**

9. Carbohydrates consist of only starch or sugar, and absolutely nothing else. **T F**

10. For nourishing muscles after exercise, you need only protein—not fat. Protein is the body's sole fuel for building muscle tissue. **T F**

The Answers

1. **False.** You should take in most of your calories during the daytime, when you can still burn them off. Eating late in the evening can pack on pounds.

2. **False.** The harder you work, the faster you lose weight. But don't work so hard that you burn out and quit.

3. **False.** Weight work burns body fat just as effectively as aerobics, in part by building new muscles, which burn extra calories.

4. **False.** Metabolic slowdown is actually extremely gradual. Don't use aging as an excuse.

5. **False.** Women really do have it harder, because estrogen can trigger body-fat storage.

6. **False.** Any movement is good—even fidgeting or pacing. Just stay active!

7. **False.** Exercise actually decreases hunger, by causing the body to produce more adrenal hormones. Only prolonged exercise, such as several hours' worth, increases hunger.

8. **False.** You should feel great after you exercise. If you're depleted, you did too much.

9. **True.** Carbs—sugar and starch—are good for providing energy only. They don't help rebuild the body.

10. **False.** Essential fatty acids—such as the EFAs found in fish—are the "vitamins of the fat world."

Your Fitness Mantra

A Personal Pep Talk

One of the smartest things you can do is to create a personal fitness mantra—a short phrase you can say to yourself at any time during the program when you need a lift.

Let's create one now.

A great way to start creating one is by taking a good, honest look at your current state of mind. To help you do this, here is a Self-Assessment Survey.

The Self-Assessment Survey

(Answer questions in the space provided.)

1. What, specifically, do I want to achieve in the next six weeks?

2. Why is my commitment to this program greater than my commitment to others I've tried?

3. Why will I succeed this time?

4. What's my biggest challenge?

5. What's my greatest motivator?

6. What's my biggest fear about fitness?

7. What's my greatest strength?

8. How can I create the time it will take to succeed with the One Body, One Life program?

9. Who am I doing this for?

10. What is the core of my support system?

Creating Your Mantra

Review your answers to the ten questions. Analyze them. What do they tell you about your goals—and your best ways of achieving them?

Now write a short, declarative statement that will help spur you to success. Such as:

"I'm doing this for myself. It's the real deal. I will never give up!"

or:

"I believe in myself. I believe in this program. This is my time to succeed."

Throughout the next six weeks—and beyond—repeat this mantra anytime you need it. Carry it in your pocket. Your mind. And your heart.

Chapter 3

The Four Elements of Fitness

Welcome to My World

I t's not your imagination: Show-business bodies really do look better than ever, because so many people in show business are exercising smarter than ever. Many of these people, I'm happy to say, are my clients. I couldn't possibly be prouder of them. They are ambitious, intelligent people who know, beyond doubt, that all of us have but one body, and one life.

And from their platform of show business, these people are challenging everybody in America to change their bodies for the better.

There is now a higher standard of fitness in America than there used to be. Fit people, in general, are more fit than they were twenty years ago.

Is that bad? I don't think so. In this current era of obesity, I wish even more people were embracing higher standards—especially America's kids, millions of whom are way out of shape.

Many of the people who are in shape, though, are in really good shape. They're part of a national revolution in smart fitness.

My pride comes from playing a role in this fitness revolution. I know that I have helped people. Many of them are people you've never heard of—just average folks. But many others are very famous.

I have, for example, helped Brad Pitt become a godlike warrior for *Troy*. I have helped

Tobey Maguire become a superhero, as Spider-Man. I've helped Leonardo DiCaprio get into absolutely peak physical condition. I've helped Pierce Brosnan do some of the things that only James Bond can do. I've helped Melanie C. transform herself into a true "Sporty Spice." I've helped Ethan Hawke move from young actor to leading man. I've helped luminous performers radiate even brighter star power: Gwen Stefani, Julianna Margulies, Rachel Weisz, and Brittany Murphy. I've helped Pink become her rockin' best. I've helped great actors, singers, and models: Ray Liotta, Kevin Spacey, Jon Bon Jovi, and Victoria's Secret's Gisele Bündchen.

They all needed different things, and I provided those things. They all changed their bodies for the better.

Now that you know about the people with whom I've worked, it's time to get down to my ideas, because it's my concepts, not my résumé, that will help you change your body.

This chapter introduces you to the four primary elements of my One Body, One Life program. All four of them work together. They are synergistic. If you put your own energy into each of the four, they will return that energy fourfold.

The Four Elements of Fitness

Element #1: Mind and Spirit

Element #2: Power Food

Element #3: Cleansing

Element #4: Exercise

Element #1: Mind and Spirit

Your mind and spirit, along with your body, are you. Therefore, if you want to be fit, your mind and spirit have to be fit.

This is not deep philosophy. This is common sense.

For your mind and spirit to be fit, you will need to address them directly. You will have to work on them, just like you work on your muscles. If you don't, they will work against you, instead of for you.

To make your mind and spirit work for you, you've got to first get over the idea that your mind controls you. The truth is, you control your mind. It is a part of you—you're not a part of it.

We often feel as if our minds run our lives—that everything starts in the brain. But that's simplistic. There's more to you than your brain.

There is a "you" in you that nobody put there—and that "you" is running your life. That "you" is your self.

Part of it was created by your brain, part was created by the events of your life, and part was created by other people. The whole you—your self—is the one that experienced these life events, experienced the workings of your own brain, and experienced the influence of other people—and then mixed this all together and somehow decided, This is me: This is my self.

If you can develop an intimate relationship with that self, you will be able to change your body—and change anything else in your life—because you will be in control of you.

You say you're a compulsive eater, and just don't have the mental strength to stop? Too many childhood traumas? Too much stress on your mind? I know you can rise above it!

You say your mind feels burned out at the end of the day, and that's why you can't get off the couch? Let's get past that. I'll help.

If you have these kinds of negative self-concepts, you just don't really know yourself yet. You don't "know your own mind."

We all have dark corners in our consciousness, but our minds are not naturally self-destructive. We are not naturally lazy. We were all born with positive mental outlooks, and with an abundance of energy. If you think your mind is overtly negative, it's because you've lost touch with your real self.

Don't worry. You can find yourself. My One Body, One Life program can help you, but mostly you'll have to help yourself. Your biggest asset in getting to know your own mind will be your spirit.

Your belief system may hold that the spirit that is inside you is part of a divine spirit, or you might think it's your own human spirit. Whatever you believe, though, you've felt your spirit, haven't you? It's ethereal—you can't touch it—but it's there. Your spirit is that amazing, mysterious part of you that's never scared and never lazy.

People call spirit many things. From my own, personal perspective, though, spirit is energy.

I love energy. It's mystical, but at the same time, plain as day. It's that special reservoir of strength that seems to somehow always stay full.

Your spirit, or energy, is also the only thing you've got that will ever give you the courage to look deeply at the dark parts of your own mind.

At this point in your life, your spirit may be hard to find, buried beneath layers of stress, and fat, and fear, and regret. I'll help you get a feel for it.

Once you get a feel for your own spirit, and get to know your own mind, you will be able to perform the important mental and spiritual feats that lead to holistic fitness.

The Aloha Spirit

As a child, I lived with my mother on the wild side of Kauai, the Garden Island of Hawaii, renowned among naturalists for its spectacular canyons and giant, vibrant flowers, and known among spiritualists as a vortex of life-force energy, or chi.

Kauai has less tourism than the other, larger islands, and partly because of this it seems to be relatively more saturated with the Aloha Spirit.

The place of your childhood always leaves an indelible stamp on you, and I'm blessed to be stamped with the Aloha Spirit.

The Aloha Spirit, more than any other single philosophy, lies at the heart of my One Body, One Life program. It is the driving, living entity that allows the stars, executives, and all of us to achieve almost superhuman results in the limited time our schedules allow.

The Aloha Spirit starts in the heart, and moves throughout the body. Here's one way of looking at it:

A	ala:	awareness
L	lokahi:	unity
O	oiaio:	honesty
H	haahaa:	humility
A	ahonui:	perseverance

In Hawaii, the kahunas, or keepers of the secrets, say that this acronym of Aloha means: "Be aware of the unity of your real self and the world around you. If you do this, you will be honest and humble, because you will know that God is inside you, and that you are inside God. But do not expect this to be easy: persevere."

Similarly, they did not see other people as being separate from themselves. They believed in the traditional Hawaiian saying: "When there is pain, it is my pain. And when there is joy, it is my joy." For them, the Aloha Spirit meant that they were a part of all, and that all was a part of them: one body, one life.

They believed that breath itself was a living being—a connection to the life force—and that each inhale brought that life force into them, and that each exhale took them into that life force.

Element #2: Power Food

Power food is fuel. You're going to learn how to fuel yourself like a Learjet. Like a Sherman Tank. You'll learn to fuel yourself for whatever kind of body you want to have.

Don't worry—your food will still taste good. It just won't have red, yellow, and blue balloons on the package. In fact, it may not come in a package.

The unalloyed truth is, all the exercise in the world won't work if you don't eat the right kind of food.

Don't you think it's weird how all these people can get on television with their "amazing" ab exercises—when the obvious key to attractive abdominal muscles is just being thin enough to see them? We've almost all got six-pack abs under there somewhere. The key to abs isn't so much how you exercise your belly, but what you put into your belly.

Like all the other main elements of fitness, learning to eat power food means getting yourself together mentally, spiritually, and physically. If your mind and spirit are unfocused and disconnected, you'll figure: I've got bigger problems right now than eating right. You can't eat right if your mental and spiritual relationship with your self is screwed up.

It's not effective enough, though, to just eat with restraint. You have to eat smart. It took me a long time to figure out smart eating, even though I had a lot of good teachers, including the Hollywood stars who monitor every bite they put into their mouths.

But eating right is not just a matter of mind power. Your body can subvert your fueling plan, too. The body has a mind of its own—literally. There are neurotransmitters all over your body, and they have elaborate relay and feedback systems with your brain. In fact, your body's largest concentration of the feel-good neurotransmitter serotonin is not in the brain, but in the nerves of your gut. Partly because of this, when you give your body the wrong fuel, it protests. Sometimes the protest is subtle, and sometimes it's screaming headaches, aching joints, and wild food cravings.

In the Power Food sections of the three phases, I'm going to dig into the details of exactly what you should eat. I'm going to help you discover the fuel that you need for your own body type, lifestyle, goals, and exercise program. You'll get the same advice from this book that you'd get if you were a superstar enrolling in my program.

Some of what I'll tell you about power eating may be new to you, because it'll be about things like food sensitivities, insulin resistance, carbohydrate intolerance, the fat-storage effects of estrogen, and food cravings.

Do you really think the stars manage to look the way they do just by eating from the four basic food groups? These people know nutrition—and you will, too.

Element #3: Cleansing

You cannot build your new body without getting rid of some of your old body. Getting fit doesn't just mean adding on to what you have. It also means subtracting: specifically, subtracting body fat and toxins.

Both of these substances are weighing you down, literally and figuratively.

Getting rid of both at once is a natural, symbiotic process, because most toxins are stored in adipose tissue, or body fat. That's part of the reason people feel better when they lose weight. They're not just freeing their bodies from the burden of an excessive load, they're also cleansing their bodies of poisons.

It doesn't feel good to carry poison in your body. It makes you feel . . . poisoned. When toxic concentration is most severe—such as from excessive inhalation of carbon monoxide—it can feel like a chronic illness. Even when toxicity is mild—from eating too many chemicalized foods, or from smoking—it can feel noticeably uncomfortable.

It's very possible that you're suffering from an uncomfortable toxic reaction right now, but just aren't aware of it. Maybe you think this is just how your body naturally feels—rather sluggish and touchy.

Your body will feel better when it's clean.

And when it does, you'll have more energy. And when you have more energy . . . well, you know the rest of the mantra by now.

If you have been living the standard American lifestyle for many years, you may have, in effect, seventy trillion garbage cans for cells. Many of your cells are probably crammed right now with necrotic debris from unassimilated foods, pesticides and herbicides, rancid fats, pollution, food dyes, drugs, secondhand smoke, and other toxins. Millions of your cells are undoubtedly dying from this.

The organs and glands in your body that eliminate toxins are probably also overloaded and backed up. Your liver may be slightly swollen, or even fatty, your kidney's nephrons may be inflamed, and your lymph glands may be so engorged with toxins that you can feel them, as some lumps. Your skin—nicknamed "the third kidney"—may be greasy, rough, and blemished from poisons that your body is trying to eliminate.

Here are just some of the conditions that are caused by excessive toxicity in the cells and tissues.

POISON PROBLEMS

- Joint pain
- Chronic cough
- Nasal congestion
- Fatigue

- Headache
- Skin blemishes
- Bad breath
- Allergies
- Inflammation
- Sore throat
- Depression
- Asthma

And here's the most common condition: You just don't feel good. Not too scientific, right? But you know the feeling I'm talking about, don't you? It feels kind of like having a hangover—but without having had the celebration first.

You cannot be fit if you're toxic. You can be brave about working out, and persevere, even when you don't feel good. Until you detoxify your cells, you just won't have the energy to make significant changes in your body. You'll never get to the next level of fitness.

Therefore, you simply must eliminate a few trillion particles of these poisons. When you do, you're going to feel like a teenager again.

My program for doing this isn't hard. A lot of people really enjoy it because they feel better almost immediately.

Cleansing is simple. It consists of avoiding toxic substances, and eliminating the ones you haven't avoided. In Phase One you'll learn how to recognize toxins and nurture your organs of elimination, and in Phases Two and Three I'll show you how to do an internal cleansing program that will make you feel great from the inside out.

I'll tell you one more thing about the cleansing program: It will help you shed pounds. How does that sound?

Element #4: Exercise

The mind and the spirit set the stage for physical fitness, but the body does the work.

That's a blessing—because work is what the body was built for. The body craves activity. To deprive it of action feels as unnatural as trying to repress thoughts in the mind.

If you think your body doesn't cherish physical activity, try not moving for a few minutes. Sit or lie perfectly still. Pretty soon, it will start to feel as if your own body is a prison.

Part of the reason activity feels good is because we're genetically programmed for it. During the evolutionary development of mankind, action equaled survival. If you sat around, you died. If you took action, you survived.

Throughout history, people just couldn't make a living without using their bodies. As recently as the early 1900s, most people in America were active for at least five to ten hours every day. Back then, 40 percent of all Americans lived on farms, and 80 percent of all farm-work was done with human labor. People who lived in towns and cities were also active, working in factories, walking wherever they went, and doing chores at home. Obesity was so uncommon that it was considered a sign of success.

Then, our society got "lucky." Progress changed everything. Now, most Americans make their livings with their minds instead of their bodies, they drive to work, and they do their chores with electrical appliances.

The good life, huh?

It's a disaster. We're dying from it.

The obesity epidemic is the modern plague. It's killing as many people—no exaggeration—as the Black Plague did in the Dark Ages (just more slowly).

But at the end of a long day, you don't have five to ten extra hours to work out, do you?

You need an approach that's built around the modern lifestyle, and geared for fast results.

It needs to be efficient. And it needs to be fun. If it's not efficient, there's no point in doing it, and if it's not fun, you won't keep it up.

I love efficiency. Time and energy are precious. If you waste either one, you're wasting part of your life. If you're not doing it right, you're not doing it.

Let me put that in boldface, so you'll notice it every time you thumb past this page:

If You're Not Doing It Right, You're Not Doing It.

You need to stay absolutely conscious during your workout. If you stay present, you'll notice every little mistake you're making, and you'll learn to do things right. When you do exercise right, two things will happen:

- **You'll gain tremendous physical power**—just like my fabulously fit clients do.
- **The appearance of your body will change.** Muscles will pop out. Flab will turn taut and tight.

If you learn to focus hard enough on the details of what you're doing, you'll be able to virtually will your muscles to grow.

And what about fun? Can't forget fun, can we? Not for you.

I know that if you're not having fun, you won't keep showing up for your workouts. That's why the first question I ask new clients is, "What do you like to do?"

Your favorite form of fitness won't be the only type of exercise that you'll do. I'll teach you how to mix it up, and keep things fresh. We're not going to stop with just some plain-vanilla lifting, stretching, and aerobics. We'll also throw in some martial arts moves, some yoga, some core interval training, Pilates—even shadow boxing. We'll go beyond cross-training, and find every muscle in your body. And we won't stop with just toning muscles. That's old-school. We'll also ignite the life force, or chi, that animates your every movement.

That's the power of exercise!

That's One Body, One Life fitness.

Part

The Three Phases *of* Fitness

Two

Chapter **4**

Phase One
The Challenge of Change

Welcome to Phase One

Today is the beginning of a major change in your body, and your life.
There will be three phases in this change, which will occur over just six weeks.

Phase One: The Challenge of Change. This phase covers weeks one and two. It's about challenge—not reward. Reward will come soon—sooner than you probably think possible.

Phase Two: Your New Body. This phase takes place during weeks three and four. By this time, due to the accelerated nature of my program, you will definitely begin to see changes in your body. You'll love it. Your motivation will soar. You'll work harder in this phase, but it will feel easier.

Phase Three: Your New Life. This phase covers weeks five and six. By this time, you will have reached a new level of power over your body. As you reach this new level, you will realize that you can't change your body without changing your life. That's good, because these changes in your life will feel great. As your body continues to improve, so will your life. If you stick with this program, you'll never be tempted to go back to your old life. It just won't feel right anymore.

The Challenge of Change

The biggest challenge of change is starting. You'll be fighting inertia, bad habits, and fear. You'll need to give everything you've got: your body, your mind, your spirit . . . and your life.

You're going to love giving this. The more you give, the more you'll get. Immediately.

In Phase One, you'll work on the Four Elements of Fitness, just as you will in Phases Two and Three. This may feel foreign at first. You may find yourself resisting. Making excuses. Cutting slack. If that happens, accept it. And move on.

Just don't quit.

I realize that change is hard, and therefore I've made Phase One as doable and realistic as possible. I don't want to lose you before you even get started.

In Phase One, you will tackle only the obstacles that I know you can overcome. We'll make this change work for you.

We'll start with basics. The fundamentals. The foundation.

The main thing is: **Just start.**

For a quick-reference guide on how this program breaks down week by week, please see Appendix D on p. 263.

Phase One | Fitness Element #1 | *Mind and Spirit*

Phase One: The Challenge of Change

Empowering Your Mind and Spirit

Your body is already quite capable of attaining fitness. Hardly anyone fails to achieve fitness due to physical problems.

The real problem, for most people, is not the body. It's the head: the mind and the spirit. If you can get your mind and spirit to embrace fitness, you will become fit.

Embracing fitness, though, means a lot more than just wanting it. Everybody wants to be fit, but that's not what makes it happen. Fitness is not only about desire. To attain fitness, you must:

- **Free yourself from fear.** Most people fail to fully embrace fitness simply because they're afraid of the work, and they're afraid they'll fail.
- **Own your body and your life.** The day you realize that you alone control your level of fitness will be the day your fitness level starts to soar.
- **Honor where you're at.** You don't improve by disliking yourself. You improve by accepting yourself.
- **Learn to focus.** Your mind is your body's greatest asset, but only if you use it. If you focus on your exercises, you'll do them right, and reap the rewards. If you just

go through the motions, you'll never change your body. If you're not doing it right, you're not doing it.

- **Find time to work out.** Your workout must become your own daily oasis, free from stress, in which you build your relationship with your self. If it's just another half-hour in the day to worry and space out, you'll never get fit. Your workout time should be your sacred time.
- **Work out for yourself.** If you work out to fulfill the desires of others, you'll eventually fail. Fitness is a relationship with self.
- **Cut no slack.** Your workout time is no time to be weak. If you cut yourself too much slack, you'll never learn how to be strong. You'll just learn all the best ways to be weak.
- **Trust your intuition.** If you overthink fitness, you'll fail. Breathe, listen, and be who you really are. Have faith in the wisdom of your "mindless mind."
- **Forget perfectionism.** It's just fear disguised as ambition.

As I've already mentioned, most of the rest of the book is written in segments, almost like short magazine pieces, instead of in solid text. The reason: I don't want you to just read a big block of text and then forget about it forever. I want you to graze on the information—piece by piece—returning repeatedly to the sections that mean the most to you.

- They'll be easy to find.
- The key concepts will be in boldface.
- The repetition of rereading them will burn the concepts into your brain.

The theme of Phase One is getting started. That means dealing with your doubts, analyzing your motivations, and then going for it.

Lose the Fear

Do you sometimes feel intimidated by exercise? Are you afraid you'll never get to where you want to go? If so, **lose the fear.**

Fear can feel like your friend, because you think it's motivating you. But all it's really doing is overwhelming you. When you get anxious, stop thinking about your whole life and your ultimate goal. Don't even think about your next challenge. Think about now. Now is never very scary. The sky is never falling right now.

If you can't stop worrying, physicalize your worry. If you're worried about getting a better butt, put your worry into your butt. Make your fear work for you, instead of against you.

I always tell people who are fighting against fear that the very best way to beat it is to just breathe. When you're expressing fear, you breathe from your chest up, or even your throat. Pull the air all the way into your root chakra—deep down below your pelvic area. That's where your warrior lives. That's where your protector is. And it needs your breath more than anywhere else.

Superstars like Brad Pitt never come from fear. When they have only a short time to transform themselves for roles, they say, "I have this challenge. I've got to get really big. What do you think?"

What do I think? I think, "Okay, let's do it!" It's easy for me to feel like that, because when somebody comes from courage, it makes everybody around them feel confident.

Tobey Maguire was fearless, even when he had the huge challenge of preparing for *Spider-Man*. He had to pack on muscle, and learn martial arts, yoga, and gymnastics. Because he is a vegetarian, hitting his protein requirements was very tough. But he never once came from fear. He just didn't invest in it. We had days when he'd wake up early, have a protein shake, do yoga, do gymnastics, take a nap, meet with producers, have another shake, and then hit the weight room. All of this in one day. He'd get a little tired, but he was always smiling. I'd look in his eyes, and they were saying, "I'm here." And my response to that was, "Well done, my friend—well done."

Learn from these people, like I did. The main illusion of fear is that it will be around forever. Fear is like a dark cloud scuttling across the sky—it never stays in one place. It's always moving. The only way fear will stay around forever is if you move with it. Let it go. Breathe it away. Blow it away.

It's not you.

It's just fear.

Your workout space is sacred. Lose the fear.

✳ AN EXERCISE FOR YOUR SPIRIT

When a fear bubbles up, take it out of your mind, take it out of your heart—and put it down on paper. Break it down. Define exactly what you're afraid of. Outline it. Almost all fear is fear of the unknown. When fear becomes known, the fear goes away. Exposed fear can become excitement. Fear and excitement live next door to each other. Knock on the door that serves you. **Take a moment to write down your worst fear about achieving fitness.**

Vanity Is Sanity
Embrace Your Desire to Look Better

Ask yourself why you are working out. And be honest.

Here are the most common reasons people want to be fit.

- To look good for a husband, wife, girlfriend, or boyfriend.
- To be fit in time for a class reunion, a wedding, a big party, or the swimsuit season.
- Your friends or family seem to have lost respect for you, and you want to regain it.

However, I hope none of these reasons are your reason. These reasons are the KISS OF DEATH for fitness.

They're all extrinsic reasons, rather than intrinsic ones. They're really about what other people want, not what you want.

Forget other people.

Other people are not going to be there with you in the Breakthrough Moment, when your muscles are burning. Their voices are not going to be inside your head, telling you how great you're doing.

Fitness is a personal matter. It's between people and their trainer (if they have one)—and nobody else. In this case, it's between you and me. Since I can't be there physically, its really between you and you. Fitness is either part of the relationship that you have with yourself—or it's nothing at all.

It's natural for people to care about each other, but if someone else has a particularly strong interest in your level of fitness, it's probably because of how it reflects upon them, rather than how it serves you. For example, if your mom or your boyfriend or your wife insists that you work out, who are they really thinking about? You? Maybe they are—if you've got a health problem that only fitness can help. More likely, though, if they're insistent enough to nag you about it, they want you to be more fit to fulfill their own needs.

This isn't cynicism, it's realism. If you want to get fit, you've got to get real.

You want to get fit to look good for your boyfriend? Bad reason.

You want to get fit to look good? Period? Good reason.

There is a difference, and you will need to recognize that difference to achieve the self-motivation required to get fit and stay fit.

Fitness is a relationship with the self. Don't ever let other people tell you what that relationship with the self should consist of. As long as your motivation is heartfelt, you should honor it, no matter what your particular motivation is.

The current trend is for fitness gurus to tell people that there's only one correct motivating factor for fitness: health. According to them, if you're not trying to improve your health you're doing it for the wrong reasons. Sorry, but I disagree. Health is not the only viable reason to get fit. What about looking sexy? That motivation might be too shallow for some people, but for most of us, it's a reasonable and laudable goal. People have been trying to look sexually attractive throughout history—and they always will. It's human nature. Vanity is sanity.

If you're a guy, maybe you want to be physically powerful because you're tired of being the one who gets sand kicked in his face. Good for you. There is nothing wrong with that motivation.

Or maybe you want to get fit for no good reason at all. Great! No reason at all can be the best possible reason. Don't overthink it. Just do it because you feel like it.

And, remember that there's no cookie-cutter motivation for fitness.

YOUR TO-DO LIST

1. Use your mantra—the one you created from the Self-Assessment Survey. Tape it to your mirror. Say it out loud.
2. Visualize yourself six weeks from now. Grab on to that image. Feed on the excitement of how good you look.
3. Find one recent improvement in yourself. Celebrate that improvement, and get caught up in the momentum of change.
4. At the end of every workout this week, focus on how good you feel. Burn that feeling into your brain.
5. Ask yourself: What's your motivation?

Focus Is the Key to Fitness

The average person likes to space out while they exercise, using loud music, a television, or just their own daydreams to take their minds off their workouts. Then they wonder why they don't get results.

That's why this is not your average fitness book.

If you want to change your body, you need to focus during your workout—not space out.

When the mind is distracted or disengaged, the body can go through the motions of exercise without really achieving much change. This happens all the time. When people do their workouts without checking in, being present, and focusing on what they're doing, they disconnect. This lack of synergy can ruin your results.

For example, people often overuse muscle groups that are already strong, simply because the body always unconsciously seeks the easiest ways to get work done. When this happens, fewer calories are burned, there is less aerobic exchange with the environment, and the muscles that are ignored continue to atrophy.

Another thing that commonly occurs when people space out during exercise is that they unknowingly cut themselves too much slack. In their mental fog, they don't realize that their heart rates aren't high enough, and they don't recognize the fact that they're working out with too little weight, speed, or intensity. It just doesn't register.

Furthermore, when people disengage mentally, they often injure themselves. They'll be vaguely aware that they're straining, and then—pop!—they'll tear a ligament or rip a muscle.

You've got to check in. Be your body. Own it.

Too boring? That only happens when you're just partly checked in. To really focus, you have to do more than just turn off the TV. You've got to engage your mind with laser-like intensity on four major elements.

1. **Establish which muscle groups you want to be working.**
2. **Determine how these muscles are feeling.** Are they exhausted or ready for more?
3. **Evaluate how you're performing the exercise.** Is it the right way or the wrong way?
4. **Decide how you want to change the muscles you're exercising.** Do you want more size, or just better tone?

If you focus on all four of these elements during each exercise, you won't have time to be bored. You will be mentally engaged.

To help yourself focus, use the mental technique of visualization. Visualize the proper performance of the exercise. Visualize how you want the muscles to look when you're done.

As you visualize, talk to yourself. Talk out loud, or silently, about how your body feels and looks, how to do the exercise properly, and how you'll feel and look when you're done.

When you focus hard—using visualization and self-talk—you will quickly enter into the nirvana of exercise: the Breakthrough Moment.

The Breakthrough Moment

The Breakthrough Moment, as I've mentioned, is that indescribably powerful state of physical being in which your muscles, in effect, are walking the razor's edge that lies between strength and utter exhaustion. In the Breakthrough Moment, you teeter on the edge of failure, because you're not sure that you can perform even one more rep. Your muscles say you can't. Your mind says you can. Who wins?

It depends. Sometimes the body, sometimes the mind. If it was a sure thing either way, it wouldn't be the Breakthrough Moment.

The Breakthrough Moment is a pure elixir of challenge, every time you enter into it.

Without focus, though, you almost never enter into it. You reflexively back off and quit, before you even approach exhaustion. Or you enlist some other muscle group to do the job, in order to escape exhaustion.

If you do focus, you can charge right into the Breakthrough Moment, where you'll often succeed at performing what I call "the golden reps."

The golden reps are the repetitions that you do in the Breakthrough Moment. When you're doing your golden reps, your muscles hurt, quiver, and cry out for respite. But these golden reps are the ones that really change your body.

You might do twenty reps of an exercise before you hit the Breakthrough Moment and get to your golden reps. If you quit before you get to the Breakthrough Moment's golden reps, though, it's very possible you won't see much change in your body. There won't be any significant growth of new muscle tissue. There may not even be much caloric expenditure.

If you regularly break into the Breakthrough Moment, into the golden reps, you're guaranteed to change your body. This is a physical fact of life.

✳ AN EXERCISE FOR YOUR SPIRIT

Practice being present. Start to notice when your mind drifts. When it does, ask yourself, "What am I thinking right now?" Get back to center by engaging with whatever you're doing. Get detailed: "I'm walking on a treadmill at 3.5 miles per hour." Physicalize your presence—feel each step you take. Feel the sides of the treadmill with your hands. Feel the gas pedal. Get out of your head and back into your body. Use your breath to connect to your core—big belly breaths. Say to yourself: "Be here. Nowhere else." Clear your mind of thought.

Do this a couple of times every day, then try to do it the next time you work out. You'll feel the difference.

Phase One | **Fitness Element #2** | *Power Food*

Phase One: The Challenge of Change

Eating Power Food

This will be the most practical, common-sense, usable info you'll ever read about nutrition. I stripped away all the hype and confusion for you, just like I do for my clients.

I have boiled down all the education I've attained about nutrition over my entire career into a single page of hard, inarguable facts.

If you can simply accept this one page of advice into your life—and live by it—all your diet problems will be over forever. That's a bold claim to make, but I can back it up in the rest of the chapter, in which I give you all the details on diet you'll ever need. Food doesn't have to be your downfall. It can be your strongest ally in your pursuit of fitness.

When you start eating right, food isn't just food anymore. It becomes power food: the prime, fundamental source of your power over your body, and your power over your life.

Everything You Ever Needed to Know about Nutrition

JUST FOLLOW THESE TWO RULES:

> **Rule #1:** Eat healthy food, in moderate portions.
> **Rule #2:** Follow Rule #1.

Definition of "healthy food": Food that is relatively low in calories and relatively high in nutrients.

Further definition of "healthy food": The food your mother told you to eat. Food that's close to the earth. Including:

- Low-fat protein (fish, beans, soy, and lean meats).
- Vegetables (especially low-starch, water-rich, high-fiber vegetables).
- Fruits.
- Whole grains, in limited amounts (particularly without added yeast).
- Foods rich in essential fatty acids (good oils, avocados, nuts).

Virtually all of this food should be whole, nonprocessed food—in other words, not in boxes.

This means you should avoid, as much as reasonably possible:

- Sugar and sweets.
- Refined grains.
- Fast food from restaurants.
- High-fat meats, trans fats, and fried foods.
- Processed foods from grocery stores.

Definition of "moderate portions": Portions that do not add up to more calories than you burn off during the day. (To learn to count calories, see "Calorie Counting," in this chapter.)

That is all you need to know.

The Long Version
of
Everything You Ever Needed to Know
about Nutrition

So you would like more details? Okay, but even this long version of the good nutrition story isn't going to be very long.

Because good nutrition is really simple.

The reasons you may think it's not simple are:

- People have tried to confuse you, in order to sell you things.
- You wanted to believe their lies, in order to find an easy way out.

The bare-bones, whole-truth, no-nonsense guideline to good nutrition is almost painfully simple. As I've said, it is: Eat healthy food, in moderate portions.

Any other approach, ultimately, will fail. Forget the gimmicks and magic. Just eat reasonable amounts of healthy food.

The ABC's of Healthy Food

There are three basic food components: protein, fat, and carbohydrates (sugar and starch), and the fundamentals of each are broken down below.

Protein

Protein should be the centerpiece of your diet. It should make up approximately 45 percent of your daily calories.

Protein is found in most foods, but is especially abundant in meat, fish, eggs, soy, dairy, beans, legumes, commercial protein powders, and nuts. You can eat abundantly from this selection of high-protein foods, as long as they don't also contain a lot of fat and carbs.

To keep your weight in control forever, you should find healthy high-protein foods that you like and base your diet around them.

Protein is important not only because it provides energy, but also because it is the only substance that rebuilds the body. Other nutrients, such as vitamins and fats, are necessary for proper biological function, and they help protein rebuild the body. However, it's protein alone that provides the building blocks that repair and replace the cells in the body. These building blocks, called amino acids, form muscle, bone, skin, organs—your entire body.

If you don't get enough protein, your body will begin to fail. Your skin will wrinkle, your organs will atrophy, and your muscles will shrivel.

Unfortunately, this type of degeneration is somewhat common, to a certain degree, among many dieters, who starve themselves of high-protein foods in order to lose body fat, but also end up losing muscle, healthy skin cells, and organ tissues.

I eat protein at virtually every meal. For breakfast, I often have a protein shake or eggs with spinach. For lunch, my main course will be a skinless chicken breast—or two, if I'm hungry. For dinner, I like to have fish, tofu, or any type of lean, quality protein. I also snack throughout the day on high-protein foods, such as yogurt or raw almonds.

Protein has a slow rate of digestion, so it really sticks to your ribs, and keeps you from getting hungry. It's great for keeping your blood-sugar levels nice and stable.

Eat low-fat, low-carb protein foods at practically every meal. That's what fit people do.

Carbohydrates

Carbs are my second highest source of calories, accounting for about 35 percent of my total caloric intake. I love carbs—starch and sugar—but I've learned to be very moderate in my consumption of them. They're too much like a drug. They sprint into your bloodstream, spike up your blood sugar and insulin, and then leave you longing for more.

I get most of my carbs from healthy, high-fiber, green vegetables, which don't destabilize blood-sugar levels because they're naturally low in carbs and calories. You should eat more servings of this type of vegetable than any other carbs in your diet. These servings, no matter how abundant, will be so low in carb calories that they will have even fewer calories than the lean proteins you eat. When you want carbs, eat veggies instead of sugar.

SUGAR

The best sugary foods are whole fruits, because even though they're sweet, they're still much lower in sugar than almost any kind of dessert or candy. Fruits also have many nutrients, and the phytochemicals that help fight disease. In addition, they're high in fiber, which helps slow the digestion of the sugar, and therefore helps prevent blood-sugar spikes.

Therefore, fruit comprises the smallest amount of my diet. Approximately 40 percent of my diet may come from carbs, but only about 5 percent of my diet is sugar.

Sugar is just fun food. It tastes great, but all it does is provide quick, temporary energy. Unlike protein, and even some fats, sugar doesn't contribute to rebuilding the body, or performing any other vital functions. It's terrible for the stability of blood-sugar levels, and it triggers hypoglycemia.

The worst kind of sugar, in my opinion, is high-fructose corn syrup, which is now the most common sugar added to processed foods. Over the past thirty years, the amount of corn syrup consumed in America has risen from one-half pound per person annually to sixty-two pounds per person. Almost all of this is corn syrup that's been added to processed foods. This increase accounts for almost 250 extra calories per person each day, which is enough to add approximately one pound of body fat every twelve days.

One of the worst things about corn syrup is that it isn't as effective as regular sugar at shutting off the brain's appetite-control mechanisms, due to its largely artificial composition. The brain doesn't fully recognize corn syrup as sugar, so people who eat it keep feeling hungry, even after they've consumed it.

One of the most common current sources of this corn syrup is soda, which people are drinking far too much of these days. Over the past thirty years, annual soda consumption has increased from about twenty-five gallons per person to approximately fifty gallons. One reason people are probably drinking more is because modern soda isn't as effective at triggering satiety as the old-fashioned, real-sugar soda was.

Bottom line:
Don't drink soda.

It's garbage. It's empty calories that don't even satisfy you.

I don't even recommend artificially sweetened soda, or other artificially sweetened foods, because the insulin system has a hard time differentiating real sweeteners from artificial sweeteners. This means that even artificial sweeteners can make blood-sugar levels fluctuate wildly.

THE OTHER CARB: STARCH

Starch really isn't much different from sugar. That's why they're both classified as carbohydrates. Pure starch rushes into the system just as quickly as sugar does, and causes similar blood-sugar swings, resulting in hunger, cravings, and energy loss.

Contrary to myth, there's no such thing as "good starch" and "bad starch," or "good carbs" and "bad carbs." Starch is starch, and a carb is a carb. But there are definitely good foods that have starch in them, and bad foods that have starch in them.

GOOD STARCHY FOODS:

- Have relatively low amounts of starch.
- Have lots of fiber.
- Have lots of nutrients.

BAD STARCHY FOODS:

- Have relatively high amounts of starch.
- Have low amounts of fiber.
- Have low amounts of nutrients.

GOOD STARCHY FOODS	BAD STARCHY FOODS
• Pumpkin	• White rice
• Apples	• White bread
• Beans	• Potatoes

Some starchy foods—particularly "white foods," like refined grains—are so full of starch, and so bereft of fiber, that they hurry into the system almost as fast as pure sugar. Following is a list of how quickly various foods enter the bloodstream. This speed is referred to as the food's glycemic index.

THE GLYCEMIC INDEX

From Fastest (or Worst) to Slowest (or Best)

1. Table sugar (Worst)
2. Instant white rice, or white rice cakes
3. White rice cereals
4. Refined breakfast cereals, from wheat or corn
5. Very sweet fruits (melon, raisins)
6. Tropical fruits
7. Brown rice
8. Whole wheat breads and crackers
9. Whole rye, pita, and pumpernickel breads
10. Unrefined, high-fiber cereals, such as bran
11. Nontropical fruits
12. Peeled vegetables
13. Unpeeled vegetables
14. Beans (Best)

Fats

Fats are the third basic food component, and comprise about 15 percent of my daily caloric intake, but I try to concentrate most of that consumption in healthy fats, rather than in unhealthy fats.

The most healthy fats are known as "essential" fatty acids, or EFAs, because they're essential for life, just like vitamins. In effect, EFAs are the vitamins of the fat world. They are found in, among other sources, many nuts and seeds, which are excellent sources of not only EFAs but also protein and fiber. These include flaxseeds, pumpkin seeds, sesame seeds, and sunflower seeds. They're great, and I eat them by the handful.

EFAs are absolutely necessary for burning body fat. That's why the protein powder that I eat has EFAs added to it. (I'll tell you where to get this special protein powder in the Phase Three section called "The Fitness Supplement A-List.") Lots of people take EFAs in pill form, as supplements, just to increase their body's abilities to burn fat.

The types of fat that I avoid are saturated fats. They're called that because they're saturated with hydrogen atoms, which make fat molecules stick together. This stickiness, unfortunately, makes them cling to the walls of your arteries. When these saturated fats work their way into your cells, it thickens the cell walls, and makes it hard for cells to function properly. Because of this, I never use saturated fats, such as margarine or lard, for cooking. Instead, I use unsaturated fats, which not only melt at room temperature, but also "melt" in the body, allowing them to be excreted normally, like other foods. The best unsaturated fats are, in order: olive oil, canola oil, flaxseed oil, soybean oil, sesame oil, and sunflower oil.

The worst type of saturated fats are hydrogenated trans fats. Sadly, one form of hydrogenated trans fat is the most popular fat in America: margarine. You should stay away from margarine. Butter is somewhat more fattening than margarine, but it's much better for you.

Meat, of course, always has fat in it, but there are huge differences in the amounts of fat. The following list shows, for example, that a six-ounce serving of light meat from turkey has only 54 fat calories (and 266 total calories), while a six-ounce serving of steak has 252 fat calories (and 458 total calories). However, they're both better than spareribs: 450 fat calories, and 702 total calories.

FAT CONTENT IN MEAT

(one serving, about 6 ounces)

		FAT CALORIES	TOTAL CALORIES
1.	Turkey, light meat	54	266
2.	Skinless chicken breast	54	284
3.	Turkey, dark meat	108	318
4.	Lean steak	126	344
5.	Chicken, dark meat	136	322
6.	Extra lean hamburger	234	450
7.	Steak	252	458
8.	Lean roast beef	306	496
9.	Lean bacon	324	436
10.	Beef rib roast	450	610
11.	Spareribs	450	702

Compare these amounts of fat, though, to the fat content and overall caloric content of fish. Obviously, fish is much lower in fat than almost any meat. The exception is salmon, which is rather high in fat—but it's all omega-3 fat, which is good for you.

FAT CONTENT IN FISH

(one serving, about 6 ounces)

		FAT CALORIES	TOTAL CALORIES
1.	Tuna, in water	18	222
2.	Shrimp	18	204
3.	Crab	36	170
4.	Scallops	122	225
5.	Clams	36	252
6.	White-type fish	72	256
7.	Oysters	108	270
8.	Salmon	162	300

The primary point here is that it's quite possible to get a great deal of low-calorie, low-fat, high-quality protein from meat or fish, if you choose the right meat or fish. Some are high in fat, but others are very moderate—especially any type of fish. To put this in perspective, three tablespoons of butter have about 327 fat calories—more than any single serving of fish, and more than a serving of many of the meats on this list.

One absolutely terrible, horrible source of fat is fast food. Take a look at the following amounts of fat calories:

FAST-FOOD FAT

		FAT CALORIES	TOTAL CALORIES
1.	McDonald's Big Mac	212	492
2.	Quarter Pounder with Cheese	244	515
3.	KFC Extra Crispy Drumsticks (3)	325	585
4.	Burger King King Size Fries	270	600
5.	Burger King Whopper	378	700
6.	Burger King Enormous Omelette Sandwich	423	730
7.	Burger King Old Fashioned Ice Cream Shake	378	1200

There's a reason critics of the fast-food industry call these foods a "Heart Attack in a Sack." The moral of the story: At a fast-food place, order the grilled chicken salad. On average, it has only about 250 to 350 total calories, with just 12 to 25 fat calories, depending on the dressing.

To recap, then, here's the breakdown of my typical daily diet:

#1	Lean Protein	45%
#2	High-fiber Carbs	35%
#3	Essential Fats	15%
#4	Fruits	5%

Most old-fashioned diet plans, such as the old government food pyramid (and even the new pyramid), call for eating more carb calories than protein calories, but that isn't appropriate for most people. It's cheap, because carbs are far less expensive than protein, but I don't think it's nearly as healthy as a moderate-protein diet. It's certainly not right for someone who works out as much as I do, and who wishes to remain in peak physical condition.

The old government pyramid, in fact, called for approximately 60 percent of the daily diet to come from carb calories. The recommendation for this large percentage contributed to the obesity epidemic that has unfolded over the past twenty-five years. Incidentally, the old pyramid's high carbohydrate ratios—which were influenced by the power of the grain industry—were very similar to those recommended by the Federal Agriculture Department in its Feedlot Guidelines for cattle.

The rest is simple. Take some supplements. Don't eat foods you're allergic to or reactive to. Limit yeast-producing foods, such as bread. Drink alcohol sparingly. Eat enough to avoid hunger. Eat for physical reasons, not emotional ones.

As you can see, there's nothing very important about food that I didn't state in the original, one-page "Everything You Ever Needed to Know about Nutrition." It still all boils down to: Eat healthy food in moderate portions. As I've said, good nutrition is simple. The only time it gets complicated is when people lie to you—in order to sell you something—or when you lie to yourself, in order to find an easy way out of eating wisely.

Of course, you're going to see or hear at least a hundred more lies about nutrition before the day is over. These lies are called commercials, and they're very persuasive. Very few of the lies will be blatant. That's too bad, because blatant lies are easy to uncover. Instead, they'll be subtly misleading. For example, ads for fast food and processed foods won't come right out and say, "Our food is very good for you." They'll say, "Our new burger is lower in fat," or they'll say, "Our new ice cream is Carb Smart." They will imply that their food has reasonable amounts of calories, and that it will make you feel good and function well. This just isn't true. You are not going to lose weight eating lots of "lite" pudding and "lo-fat" potato chips. It won't happen.

Nobody in the food industry is going to be honest with you—so you've got to be honest with yourself. Painfully honest. If you are honest, a whole new world of possibilities will open up.

You will take control of your eating habits. You'll take control of your body. And, with any luck at all, you'll take control of your life.

✳ AN EXERCISE IN NUTRITION

Right now, be your own nutritionist. Create a one-day menu plan based on your own best interests, instead of your favorite foods. Be realistic. Be honest. You know intuitively what foods serve you best. Don't think of this menu as a temporary weight-loss diet. Think of it as the eating plan for the rest of your life. Then put it away until the end of the program. What you'll probably find is that this plan—which may seem challenging now—will fit the new you perfectly.

Calorie Counting

To be thin and fit, you don't really need to know many details about nutrition. All you really need to know is this:

**At the end of the day,
what matters most is calories in vs. calories out.**

Therefore, the rock-bottom foundation of weight management is knowing how many calories are in various foods.

But keep it simple.

You don't need to memorize tables. You just need to get a feel for which foods are high-calorie and which are low-calorie.

When you learn this, it will hammer home these two vital points:

- **You can eat low-calorie foods until you're completely satisfied, and still lose weight.**
- **You can only eat high-calorie foods in very small amounts.**

This is an absolute fact of life. It should be carved in stone. But it's amazing how many people don't really get it.

How Many Calories Can I Eat?

Before you learn to count calories, you should first get a sense of how many calories you can eat without gaining weight.

Here's a simple but effective way to calculate it.

- **Active people:** Multiply your weight by 15. That's the number of calories you can eat every day without gaining weight. (Example: 150 pounds times 15 equals 2,250 calories per day.)
- **Moderately active people:** Multiply your weight by 13 (at 150 pounds, 1,950 calories).
- **Inactive people:** Multiply your weight by 11 (at 150 pounds, 1,650 calories).

This number of calories should keep you from gaining weight, but it won't allow you to lose weight.

Let's say you want to lose about one pound of body fat per week. That's a very reasonable rate of weight loss, and will not trigger the starvation effect of caloric hoarding and result in a rebound weight gain. To lose one pound of body fat, you need to eliminate about 3,000 calories, through food restriction or extra exercise. If you do it with food restriction, divide 3,000 calories by seven days, which is 428 calories per day. Therefore, subtract 428 calories from your daily total. (Example: if you're an active 150-pound person, you can eat 2,250 calories, so subtract 428 from 2,250. It comes to 1,822 calories per day.)

If you choose to lose weight with extra exercise instead of food restriction, you should know that exercise burns about 300 to 500 calories per hour, depending on how strenuous it is. Jogging, for example, burns about 500 calories per hour, and walking burns about 250.

Therefore, when you combine caloric restriction with exercise—and empower these two elements with cleansing and mental focus—the sky's the limit!

The next step is to count calories. I've categorized foods from the lowest-calorie foods to the highest, and assigned each group a grade: "A+" through "F." Let's start with foods that are so low in calories that you can eat them until they come out your ears. These are the A+ foods. They're followed by the A foods and the A− foods. These foods should make up the bulk of your diet. Grade B and C foods should be consumed in moderation, and grade D and F foods should be avoided.

Calorie Grade: A+ Low-calorie, Water-rich, High-fiber, Low-starch Vegetables

These veggies are so high in fiber and water content, and low in starch calories, that you can eat virtually all you want of them and never get fat. You could—no exaggeration—eat about five servings at every meal. Vegetables are also packed with cortenoids, which are antioxidants—supplying phytochemicals.

All portions are 1 cup, raw.

FOOD	CALORIES
Asparagus	30
Bamboo shoots	42
Bell peppers	40
Bok choy	10
Broccoli	24
Cabbage (all types)	18
Carrots	48
Cauliflower	26
Celery	20
Collard greens	12
Cucumbers	14
Eggplant	22
Green beans	34
Kale	34
Leek	64
Lettuce (all types)	8
Mushrooms	18
Onions	60
Radish	20
Spinach	12
Sprouts—alfalfa, bean, mungbean, snow pea	25
Snow peas	60
Tomato	38
Yellow squash	24
Zucchini	18

Calorie Grade: A+   Low-calorie, High-protein Fish

You can eat almost as much fish as you wish without getting fat. Considering the high amount of protein it packs, it's extraordinarily low in calories. Salmon has some caloric fat, but it's good, omega-3 fat. Fish also has a very high satiety rating.

All portions are 6 ounces, raw.

FOOD	CALORIES
Clams	252
Crab	170

FOOD	CALORIES
Halibut	239
Lobster	280
Oysters	270
Pollack	192
Salmon	241
Scallops	150
Sea bass	211
Shrimp	180
Snapper	169
Tilapia	171
Trout	202
Tuna (in water)	240

Calorie Grade: A— Lean Meat: Moderate Calories, Good Satiety, Great Protein

Lean meat is so filling and nutritious that it's well worth its moderate caloric load. But it's got to be lean. For fatty meats, you can basically double these numbers. Stay away from fatty meats. You'll note that I also added eggs, beans, and tofu to this category.

All portions are 6 ounces, unless otherwise noted, and raw.

FOOD	CALORIES
Beef burger, extra lean	397
Beef steak, lean without fat	370
Chicken breast (skinless)	240
Eggs (2)	150
Egg whites (2)	90
Ham, lean	375
Lentils (1/2 cup)	115
Lima beans (1/2 cup)	104
Pork, sirloin, lean without fat	402
Red kidney beans (1/2 cup)	112
Tofu	188
Turkey breast (skinless)	150
Veal, sirloin, lean without fat	286
Vegetarian burger	150

Calorie Grade: A— Moderate-calorie, High-starch Vegetables

There's a big difference between low-starch and high-starch vegetables. Even so, high-starch vegetables can still be eaten in relative abundance.

All portions are 1 cup.

FOOD	CALORIES
Corn	136
Peas	160
Potato	140
Sweet potato	160

Calorie Grade: A— Essential Fats: Great Nutritional Value, Moderate Calories

Good fats do exist, and they are known as the essential fatty acids: Omega-3 and omega-6 are the healing fats, and every cell in your body needs them for overall health. These help the body burn fat by increasing the production of a certain group of prostaglandins or eicosanoids. I want you to add these foods to your home, pronto!

All portions are noted.

FOOD		CALORIES
SEEDS (RAW)		
Linseed (flaxseed)	(1 tablespoon)	37
Pumpkin seeds	(1 tablespoon)	77
Sesame seeds	(1 tablespoon)	24
Sunflower seeds	(1 tablespoon)	93
OILS		
Flaxseed oil	(1 tablespoon)	120
Olive oil (extra virgin cold pressed)	(1 tablespoon)	120
Sesame oil, toasted	(1 tablespoon)	120
EXTRA FATS		
Almond butter	(1 tablespoon)	97
Almonds (raw)	6	45
Avocado	(2 tablespoons)	60
Olives	4	25

Calorie Grade: A— Low-calorie, High-nutrition Fruits

Fruits are so sweet that they're suitable as desserts, but they're still quite low in calories, and high in fiber and nutrients.

All portions are 1 cup unless noted, and raw.

FOOD	CALORIES
Apples	162
Bananas	208
Blackberries	74
Blueberries	82
Cantaloupe	58
Cherries	78
Cranberries	46
Grapefruit	74
Lemon (1)	44
Lime (1)	20
Mango	108
Oranges	78
Peaches	74
Pears	98
Plums	92
Raspberries	62
Strawberries	46
Watermelon	50

Calorie Grade: B Dairy: Relatively High Calories, Good Nutrition

If you're not lactose intolerant, low-fat dairy can be good, in modest portions. It's high in protein, but is generally not as nutritious as fish or lean meat. You'll note that I also added non-dairy to this category.

All portions are 1 cup unless noted.

FOOD	CALORIES
Cheddar cheese (shredded, low fat)	320
Cottage cheese (low fat)	180
Cream cheese, light	400
Milk (2%)	121
Mozarella cheese (shredded, low fat)	280
Nondairy cheese	320
Ricotta cheese (low fat)	200
Soy milk, low carb	100
Soy yogurt, plain (nonfat)—probiotic	240
Yogurt, plain (nonfat)—probiotic	120

Calorie Grade: C   Grains: Moderate Calories, Fair Nutrition

Grains can be dangerous to your diet, especially if they're processed. They're metabolized quickly, and can spike insulin. Whole grains have some good nutrients, particularly without added yeast and saturated fat, but it's easy to eat too much of them.

All portions are 1 cup unless noted.

FOOD	CALORIES
WITHOUT ADDED YEAST:	
Non-yeast wheat-free crackers–Ryvita (5)	175
Non-yeast wheat-free crackers–Kavli (5)	100
Non-yeast wheat-free crackers–Wasa Light Rye (5)	125
Sprouted bread (1 slice)	140
WITH YEAST AND SATURATED FAT:	
Bagel (1)	90
Bread (1 slice)	65
Tortilla chips	139

Calorie Grade: D   Sweets: Too Many Calories—Poor Nutrition

Sweets must be limited in your diet if you want to see results.

All servings are 1 cup unless noted.

FOOD	CALORIES
Apple pie (1 piece)	280
Brownie	290
Chocolate fudge cake (1 piece)	310
Doughnut, plain (1)	170
Ice cream	320

Calorie Grade: F   High-sugar, High-fat Processed Foods and Fast Foods

These foods do not serve you, and should be eliminated from your diet.

All servings are 1 cup unless noted.

FOOD	CALORIES
Cheese puffs (5 ounces)	800
Cookies (4)	500
Croissant (1)	235
Double hamburger (fast food)	640
Fish sandwich (fast food)	488
French fries	300
Fried chicken (2 pieces)	480
Mayonnaise (3 tbsp.)	300
Onion rings	274
Pizza (3 slices)	625
Taco (fast food)	619

Nutrition Guidelines: Creating Your Daily Meal Plan from Each Category of Food

PROTEIN

- Always start your meal with a mouthful of protein.
- Have 3 servings of protein from the protein lists each day.
- Try to get most of your protein from the grade A+ protein list.
- Do not have more than 2 eggs a day.
- Do not have beans more than twice a week, limit ½ cup at each serving.
- Do not have cheese more than once a day, limit ¼ cup daily.
- Do not have yogurt more than once a day, limit 1 cup daily.

VEGETABLES

- Along with your protein, the bulk of the meals should be obtained from water-rich fibrous vegetables from the grade A+ list.
- Have a minimum of 5 servings of vegetables from the daily vegetable list.
- You may have the same vegetables more than once; they are interchangeable.
- Exception: Limit carrots, tomatoes, and onions to ½ cup a day.
- Exception: Limit high-starch vegetables from the grade A− list to ½ cup a day.

ESSENTIAL FATS

- Include all four seeds from the list, 1 to 2 tablespoons each day.
- Include 1 tablespoon of oil each day, cold and never heated.
- Include 2 servings of extra fat from almonds, almond butter, avocado, or olives daily.
- No margarine, hydrogenated vegetable oils, or trans fats allowed.

FRUITS

- Have 2 fruits per day from the fruit list; one of these must be an apple.
- Exception: lemons and limes.
- Only fresh or frozen fruit allowed, organic if possible; absolutely no canned fruit allowed.

WHOLE GRAINS

- Limit whole grains to 5 wheat, yeast, and fat-free crackers or 1 slice of sprouted wheat-free bread each day.

HERBS, SPICES, AND CONDIMENTS

- There is no restriction on fresh-dried herbs and spices.
- No premixed spices like barbeque or chicken spices allowed.
- No table salt allowed; use sea salt instead.
- No condiments are allowed except for 1–2 teaspoons of organic ketchup, 1–2 teaspoons of whole grain mustard, 1–2 teaspoons of tamari and Tabasco to taste.

Study **these lists and guidelines, and stick them on your fridge.** The patterns are obvious. You can eat healthy foods in abundant, satisfying quantities, and never be hungry or fat. If you eat the wrong foods, you'll never fill up, you'll never feel good, and you'll never, ever get thin.

✳ AN EXERCISE IN NUTRITION

Keep a journal of your eating. Get it out of your head and onto paper. Write down not only what you eat, but also how much, and when. Notice the patterns. Are they healthy? If you're not satisfied with what you see, ask yourself why. What are the portion sizes? Is there an excess of sweets? Are you eating too late at night, or too much comfort food?

You might find that a few little tweaks here and there will create fantastic changes.

Make your list visible. Tape it to your mirror or fridge. Don't hide from it. Embrace it. Own who you are. Love who you are.

And, when in doubt, reread the Power Food section.

SAMPLE DAILY MENU

Lean but Healthy
1,650 Calories

BREAKFAST

Glass of lukewarm water squeezed with 1 medium lemon   22

Egg Scramble with Herbs:
1 egg   75
4 oz egg whites   60
1/2 cup onions, cooked   47
1/2 cup green bell pepper, cooked   19

Side of Spinach:
1 cup boiled/steamed spinach   42
2 tbsp sesame seeds   48

DURING EXERCISE

Fat Burning Lemonade Mixed in Water:
2 scoops Fat Burning Lemonade   20
8 oz water   0

SNACK

Fruit Topped with Yogurt and Seeds:
1/2 cup strawberries, fresh   23
1 apple, chopped   81

1 cup plain unsweetened soy yogurt   120

1 tbsp sunflower seeds   93

1 tbsp pumpkin seeds   77

2 tbsp linseed (flaxseed)   74

2 non-yeast wheat-free crackers (Ryvita)   70

LUNCH

Grilled Chicken Breast:

4 oz chicken breast (skinless), cooked   160

Side of Greek Salad:

1 cup lettuce   0

$1/2$ cup onions, raw   30

$1/2$ cup tomatoes, raw   19

$1/2$ cup cucumber, raw   0

4 olives   25

1 tbsp olive oil or flaxseed oil   120

SNACK

Side of Non-Yeast Wheat-Free Crackers and Spread:

3 non-yeast wheat-free crackers (Kavli)   60

2 tbsp avocado   60

DINNER

Fish:

4 oz snapper, steamed or baked (spray with olive oil)   145

Side of Steamed Cauliflower and Broccoli Topped with Cheese:

1 cup cauliflower   14

1 cup broccoli   22

$1/4$ cup mozzarella shredded low-fat cheese   140

SNACK

6 almonds   45

COMMENTS:

This menu plan is quite low in calories—only about 1,700 per day—but still provides abundant nutrition. When you eat only healthy, wholesome whole foods, you can enjoy a satisfying diet while still losing weight.

SAMPLE DAILY MENU

To Be Slim without Suffering
1,850 Calories

BREAKFAST

Glass of lukewarm water squeezed with 1 medium lemon   22

Fruit Salad Topped with Yogurt and Cinnamon:
1 apple, chopped   81
$^1/_2$ cup strawberries, fresh   26
1 cup plain unsweetened soy yogurt   120
cinnamon (assists in glucose stability)   0

Side of Non-Yeast Wheat-Free Crackers and Spread:
3 non-yeast wheat-free crackers (Wasa light rye)   75
2 tbsp avocado   60

supplements: 1 × omega-3 oil, 1 × calcium, 1 × multivitamin, 1 × Immune Elixir   10

DURING EXERCISE

Fat Burning Lemonade Mixed in Water:
2 scoops Fat Burning Lemonade   20
8 oz water   0

SNACK

Toasted Trail Mix:

Toast on low heat:

6 almonds   45
1 cup plain unsweetened soy yogurt   120
1 tbsp sunflower seeds   93
1 tbsp pumpkin seeds   77
2 tbsp linseed (flaxseed)   74
2 tbsp sesame seeds   48
1 tsp tamari, low sodium, or sea salt   0

LUNCH

Sliced Turkey:

4 oz turkey breast (skinless) cooked and sliced   100

Side of Green Salad:

1 cup lettuce   12
1/4 cup shallots, sliced   8
1/2 cup tomatoes, sliced   19
1/2 cup cucumber, sliced   7
1/2 cup carrots, grated   24
4 olives   25

Dressing:

1 tbsp olive oil or flaxseed oil   120
3 tsp whole-grain mustard   10
1/2 tsp sea salt   0

SNACK

Cream Cheese Dip and Vegetables:

1/4 cup light cream cheese   100
hint of chili powder   0

Vegetables:

Boil one to three minutes, drain, plunge in ice water, drain, and pat dry:

1 cup carrots (cut into sticks)   70
1 cup celery (cut into sticks)   20
1 cup asparagus   44
1/2 cup broccoli   22
1/2 cup green beans   22

DINNER

Grilled Scallops and Shrimp with Garlic and Herbs:

4 oz scallops   100
4 oz shrimp   112
2 tsp garlic, minced   26
mixed herbs   0

Side of Steamed Asparagus:

1 cup asparagus   44

supplements: 1 × omega-3 oil, 1 × calcium, 1 × Immune Elixir   10

SNACK

Non-Yeast Wheat-Free Crackers with Sliced Egg:

2 non-yeast wheat-free crackers (Ryvita)   70

1 egg, boiled   75

$^1/_2$ tsp sea salt   0

COMMENTS:

This menu is only about 1,850 calories. Even a moderately active 160-pound person could lose weight eating this food. But this one-day menu doesn't seem like a typical weight-loss diet, does it? That's because it consists of healthy foods in moderate portions. When you eat the right foods, you can have an abundance of volume, and still stay at a low-calorie level.

SAMPLE DAILY MENU

For Building Lean Muscle with a Vegetarian Diet
1,950 Calories

BREAKFAST

Glass of lukewarm water squeezed with 1 medium lemon   22

Breakfast Shake:

Blend the following ingredients:

$^1/_2$ cup strawberries, frozen   26

1 scoop protein powder (protein complete organic whey)   120

1 oz unsweetened cranberry juice   10

8 oz water   0

supplements: 1 × omega-3 oil, 1 × calcium   10

DURING EXERCISE

Fat Burning Lemonade Mixed in Water:

2 scoops Fat Burning Lemonade   20

8 oz water   0

Side of Non-Yeast, Wheat-Free Crackers and Spread:

2 non-yeast wheat-free crackers (Ryvita)   70

1/2 tbsp almond butter   37

LUNCH

Carrot and Ginger Soup, Topped with Seeds:

Boil (vegetable broth for soup):

1 cup celery   0

1/2 cup onion   47

1 cup mushroom   42

4 cloves garlic   0

parsley, bay leaves   0

8 oz water   0

Strain and discard vegetables, and retain broth.

Steam:

2 cups carrots   70

1 inch ginger   0

Blend together with broth.

Dry roast:

1 tbsp sunflower seeds   93

1 tbsp pumpkin seeds   77

2 tbsp sesame seeds   48

1 tbsp linseed (flaxseed)   74

Add to soup.

Steamed Tofu:

4 oz tofu   80

Side of Marinated Raw Kale:

2 cups kale · 84

1 medium lemon (juiced)   22

1 tbsp olive oil   120

2 tsp garlic (minced)   0

1 tsp sea salt   0

SNACK

Fruit Topped with Yogurt and Cinnamon:

1 apple, chopped   81

1 cup plain, unsweetened soy yogurt   120

cinnamon (assists in glucose stability)   0

DINNER

Two Grilled Veggie Burgers:

8 oz veggie burger, Morning Star, grilled   265

Spray with olive oil spray.

Egg Salad:

1 egg, chopped   75

1 cup spinach, raw (loose baby spinach)   42

$1/2$ cup tomatoes, raw   19

$1/2$ cup cucumber, raw   0

1 tbsp olive oil or flaxseed oil   120

supplements: 1 × omega-3 oil, 1 × calcium   10

SNACK

Side of Non-Yeast, Wheat-Free Crackers and Spread:

3 non-yeast wheat-free crackers (Ryvita)   105

2 tbsp avocado   60

COMMENTS:

To help prepare a vegetarian client for building lean muscle and at the same time trimming up, we needed to increase the protein intake but keep the calories low. By adding high-protein foods, though, we created a diet that was still vegetarian but exceptionally rich in muscle-building amino acids, and was only about 2,000 calories.

SAMPLE DAILY MENU

For Building Lean Muscle with a Non-Vegetarian Diet
2,300 Calories

BREAKFAST

Glass of lukewarm water squeezed with 1 medium lemon   22

1 egg, boiled   75
1/2 tsp sea salt   0

Side of Grilled Tofu:
4 oz tofu (spray with olive oil)   80
1/2 tsp sea salt   0

Side of Non-Yeast Wheat-Free Crackers and Spread:
3 non-yeast wheat-free crackers (Wasa light rye)   75
2 tbsp avocado   60

supplements: 1 × omega-3 oil, 1 × calcium, 1 × multivitamin, 1 × Immune Elixir   10

DURING EXERCISE

Fat Burning Lemonade Mixed in Water:
2 scoops Fat Burning Lemonade   20
8 oz water   0

SNACK

Blueberry Shake:

Blend the following ingredients:

1/2 cup blueberries, frozen   50
1 scoop protein powder (protein complete organic whey)   120
1 oz unsweetened cranberry juice   10
8 oz water   0

Vegetable Crudités:

Boil one to three minutes, drain, plunge in ice water, drain, and pat dry:

1 cup carrots (cut into sticks)   70
1 cup celery (cut into sticks)   20
1 cup asparagus   44
1/2 cup broccoli   22
1/2 cup green beans   22

Bean Dip:

Blend:

1/2 cup red kidney beans   112
1/4 cup light cream cheese   100
1/4 cup water   0
1 tsp garlic, minced   0
1 tbsp parsley, minced   0
1/2 medium lemon, squeezed   11
sea salt and a hint of chili   0

Non-Yeast Wheat-Free Crackers and Spread:

2 non-yeast wheat-free crackers (Ryvita)   70

SNACK

Vegetable Juice:
2 cups carrot   48
2 cups celery   40
1 cup spinach   42
1/2 medium apple   40
ginger (optional)   0

DINNER

Thai Salmon Burger with Almond Butter Sauce:

Chop and blend with food processor:

6 oz salmon fillet (skinned)   351
1/4 cup onions   24

2 tsp ginger, freshly grated   0
1 tsp tamari, low sodium   0

Almond Butter Sauce:

Blend:

1 tbsp almond butter, raw   75
2 tsp tamari, low sodium   0
$^1/_2$ medium lemon, squeezed   11
1 tsp garlic, minced   0

Side of Cucumber:
1 cup cucumber (peeled), chopped   14

Slaw Salad:
1 cup red cabbage (raw), thinly sliced   34
1 cup green cabbage (raw), thinly sliced   34
$^1/_2$ cup carrots (raw), grated   24
$^1/_2$ cup snow peas (raw), thinly sliced   30
2 tbsp sesame seeds   48
$^1/_2$ cup green onion/scallions (raw), thinly sliced   16

Dressing:
1 tbsp sesame oil, toasted   120
$^1/_2$ tsp ginger, freshly grated   0

supplements: 1 × omega-3 oil, 1 × calcium, 1 × Immune Elixir   10

SNACK

Apple Topped with Yogurt and Seeds:
$^1/_2$ medium apple   40
1 cup plain, unsweetened soy yogurt   120
1 tbsp sunflower seeds   93
1 tbsp pumpkin seeds   77
1 tbsp linseed (flaxseed)   74

COMMENTS:
This is an ambitious diet to get in peak physical condition and requires high physical output. Note the diet's reliance upon lean meat, fish, and fresh vegetables, which keep it low in calories. This diet is about 2,300 calories per day.

Phase One: The Challenge of Change

Cleansing Your Body of Toxins

Cleansing is the element of fitness nobody ever talks about. I don't know why. It's vitally important. I think that most fitness experts simply don't know much about it. They tend to focus myopically on hard-core body-image issues, such as body-fat percentage and muscle strength. They usually don't pay enough attention, however, to the important, holistic health forces that impact these body-image issues, such as general health, energy levels, and mood.

Health, energy, and a positive mood—which are absolutely essential for achieving long-term fitness—depend upon several major factors. One of the most important of these factors is toxicity.

Our bodies are constantly exposed to a barrage of toxins, and these toxins can wreak irrevocable harm upon health, energy, and mood. They can single-handedly destroy even the best fitness programs.

Many of the toxins that invade our bodies come straight from the environment—from air pollution, water pollution, and exposure to chemicals. Even more come from the foods we eat, which are often tainted with pesticides, herbicides, food dyes, and rancid fats. Other toxins come from alcohol, cigarettes, recreational drugs, and even the pharmaceutical drugs that we take to stay healthy. Still others are macrotoxins, such as yeast overgrowth and parasites.

Most toxins are stored in adipose tissue, or fat cells. They also become lodged in the cells that compose our organs of elimination—including the liver, kidneys, and colon—and in other cells throughout our bodies. Organs of elimination are designed to expel toxins.

Stored toxins often cause obvious, notable damage to the organs of elimination. Many people have livers that are swollen or kidneys that are inflamed. You've probably frequently experienced swelling in your lymph glands, which collect toxins for elimination. Innumerable people also have small pockets in the walls of their colons, due to toxic overload and improper elimination. These pockets, called diverticula, can easily become infected, causing diverticulitis.

The fact of the matter is, the human body is made up of about seventy trillion cells, and if you have been living a conventional American lifestyle for a number of years, you may now have, as I've mentioned, seventy trillion garbage cans for cells.

That's a dire assessment, but it's realistic. After all, approximately 25 percent of the U.S. population dies from cancer, and cancer is frequently related to toxins from cigarettes, foods, chemicals, air pollution, and other sources. Toxins also cause a wide range of other, less serious problems—everything from allergies to asthma, and skin rashes to swelling.

Toxins frequently cause the most uncomfortable symptoms when they are dislodged from cells and are in the process of being eliminated from the system. They can overwhelm the organs of elimination, and begin to circulate once again in the bloodstream. This can cause headaches, sore gums, skin blemishes, fatigue, a coat on the tongue, lung congestion, watery eyes, itching, and mood swings.

Because most toxins are stored in fat cells, losing weight can cause a mass exodus of toxins from the body. That's good! It's one of the best things about eliminating body fat. But it usually doesn't feel good. It can actually make you feel pretty miserable. Many people who lose weight aren't aware that they're expelling toxins, and they think that the process of weight loss itself is intrinsically uncomfortable. Sometimes, this flushing away of toxins makes people feel so bad that they go off their diets, or cut back on exercise. This stops the breakdown of fat cells, stops the egress of toxins, and temporarily relieves the negative symptoms. People think, "That feels better—I guess losing weight is just too painful to be worth it." And that's the end of their commitment to fitness.

It's not necessary.

There are several important methods of relieving toxic overload, and of empowering the organs of elimination, so that they can get rid of toxins as quickly as the toxins arrive.

This section is all about how to do that.

It's simple stuff—just as so many of the primary elements of health and fitness are simple. It includes sweating toxins out of the skin, pushing them out of the gastrointestinal tract with extra fiber, and clearing them from the urinary tract with extra water and juices.

These techniques are easy but important. Once you start using some of them, you'll become practically addicted to them, just as you can get addicted to healthy food. This addiction comes from an almost irresistible force: pleasure. Doing it feels better than not doing it.

One of these detoxification methods is a full-scale, all-out attack on toxins that I call the Weekend Cleansing Program. It lasts for one day in Phase Two, and two days in Phase Three. When you do it, you'll feel as if your world has expanded, and everything around you is a little bit brighter and lighter. It's like a clean slate. A fresh start. You'll have more mental clarity, more spiritual focus, and more physical power. You won't be able to wait to hit the gym, or to go to the beach for a long walk.

Believe me, there's nothing like the feeling you get when you cleanse your body of toxins. Let us begin.

The following is a list of conditions associated with toxicity:

Gallstones	Eczema	Cirrhosis
Headaches	Acne	Chronic fatigue syndrome
Gastritis	Vaginitis	Abscesses
Bronchitis	Alzheimer's disease	Rheumatoid arthritis
Emphysema	Depression	Constipation

High blood pressure	Prostatitis	Cervical dysplasia
Hepatitis	Kidney stones	Pancreatitis
Diverticulitis	Parasites	Bloating
Sinusitis	Peptic ulcers	Hives
Irritable bowel syndrome	Diarrhea	Nausea

✳ AN EXERCISE IN CLEANSING

Circle the conditions on this list that have caused you problems. If there are more than three or four, you probably suffer from excess toxicity. If you do, read all of the cleansing sections in this book very carefully, and weave their advice into the fabric of your life. You'll feel reborn.

The Phase-One Cleanse

In each of the three phases, you engage in a cleansing regimen. In Phase One, you start your cleansing regimen in the most accessible way, by focusing on getting an abundance of pure air and pure water into your system. What could be easier than breathing and drinking water, or more important?

Pure water is the elixir of life. Fresh air is the breath of life.

These two most basic elements of life trigger the body's own powers of detoxification and restoration. They jump-start the cleansing process.

- They will help you achieve more energy.
- They will help rid your body of toxins stored deep in cells.
- They will help you lose weight, by sparking your vitality.
- They will dramatically improve your cognitive function.

Water: The Elixir of Life

Improbable as it may sound, water intake plays a major role in the metabolic process of burning body fat. Therefore, you should follow this basic rule:

**Drink half your weight—in ounces—each day.
For example: If you weigh 200 pounds,
drink 100 ounces of water each day.**

To make this amount easy to visualize, remember that 100 ounces would be about the same as eight 12-ounce bottles.

As part of this fluid intake, you may wish to drink two servings daily of Fat Burning Lemonade™, a very healthy product that's described in detail in the Phase Three section entitled "The Fitness Supplement A-List." A good time to drink this lemonade is while you're exercising, to help your body convert fat to energy.

To add a little variety to your fluid intake, you may enjoy drinking pure, unsweetened fruit juice. Juice can be high in calories, so it's wise to dilute it with water. A particularly good juice is cranberry juice, which is a mild diuretic and a great nutrient for the health of the urinary tract. Drink it unsweetened (without corn syrup), and mix it with water, to reduce the calories.

When you begin to use water as an important part of your training program, you'll find that:

- Water naturally suppresses the appetite. Many overweight people mistake thirst for hunger.
- Drinking lots of water actually helps you lose water-weight. That's ironic, but true. The more you drink, the more you trigger natural elimination.
- Water helps the body create muscle tissue. If you don't replace fluids after a workout, you lose much of the value of exercise.

Water is the single most essential component of all living things. Your brain is 76 percent water. Your lungs are 90 percent water. Your blood is 84 percent water. Critical physical processes—such as digestion, circulation, muscle building, and elimination—are severely compromised if fluid intake is too low. Water carries nutrients to all body tissues, plays a crucial role in regulating body temperature, and is a major element in the growth and repair of the body.

Huge volumes of toxic material are excreted every single day by your kidneys. Make the most of this natural process. You'll feel the difference.

Oxygen: The Breath of Life

Breathing is often an underappreciated component of health and fitness. It literally provides the spark of life to every cell in the body. When breathing is too shallow, it starves the cells of energy. This type of inadequate breathing subverts the functions of the major organs, hampers energy, slows down the thinking processes, and even wrinkles the skin. It keeps toxins stuck exactly where they are.

Therefore, one of the most important things you can do in Phase One is to become aware of your breathing.

- Focus on breathing from your belly, instead of just the top of your chest.
- Stop yourself from inhaling quick, tense little gulps of air that don't "feed the fire" of your energy.
- Consciously use your breath to control your stress. Do it practically every time you start to stress out.

Best of all, start using some yoga breathing techniques. Yoga revolves around breathing. Start with the simplest steps:

1. Observe your breath. Breathe in and out evenly, through your nose. In yoga, this is called *samavrtti* breathing.
2. Notice where your breath is. Determine if it comes too often from your chest instead of your belly.
3. Feel your breath physically, by placing your hand on your belly.
4. Visualize your breath. Mentally observe it as it fills your core and feeds your body.

Here are two more breath exercises for you to do in Phase One. Practice them each day.

Kumbhaka Breathing

Relax your chest and belly, and take a good, deep breath as you count slowly to four. Hold it for a moment. Then exhale slowly, until your lungs feel totally empty. Hold the exhale for a moment. Then take another deep breath, and hold it. Stick out your tongue, close your eyes, and let your breath out forcefully, as you make a powerful sound, such as "Agghhhh!" Feel the tension leave your body.

Repeat the process at least one more time.

Ujjayi Breathing

This yoga breathing technique, pronounced *ooh-jah-yee*, is also called the Breath of Victory. When you focus your mind as you do it, it brings you to a deeper sense of your selfhood. It's also a great way to warm your body, bring blood to your internal organs, and expel toxins through the breath.

To do it, simply breathe in and out through your nose, focusing on pushing and pulling the air with the back of your throat. As you do this, you will create a resonant sound, almost like snoring, as your breath rolls up and down your throat.

If you do some *ujjayi* breathing early in the morning, it's a great time to set your intentions for the day. What do you want to happen? Create your vision of the day ahead. Make it happen.

You should start your new emphasis on cleansing your body, mind, and spirit in Phase One—with an abundance of pure water and fresh air—and then continue it into Phases Two and Three. By then, it will be a part of you—because it feels so good. And it will stay a part of you.

Phase One | Fitness Element #4 | *Exercise*

Phase One: The Challenge of Change

Using the Power of Exercise

Your body is hungry for exercise. The body craves physical activity just as much as it craves air and water.

I want you to start exercising today—if you haven't already started. You should read some, or all, of the written material on exercise, which follows immediately—but even if you don't get through all of it, it's time to get physical. Skip ahead to the back of the book, where you'll find the workouts, and start working.

What's Your Fitness IQ?

ROUND TWO

Answer "true" or "false" for each question.

1. As a general rule, the more you exercise, the greater your appetite is and the more you naturally tend to eat. So weight loss from exercise is often slower than many people expect.   **T F**

2. People who try to lose weight from exercise should realize that when you end your exercise program, newly developed muscle tissue can degenerate into adipose tissue, or fat. This is an excellent reason to never stop exercising.   **T F**

3. Focusing exercise on an overweight problem area will help concentrate your weight loss on that area. This is not only common sense, but is in accord with the latest research. **T F**

4. You get the same essential benefits from exercising in four 15-minute segments, spread throughout the day, that you get from exercising for one hour straight. **T F**

5. The primary reason that women tend to gain weight more readily than men is because, in general, their professional lives and recreational lives are somewhat more sedentary. To blame it on other, supposedly uncontrollable forces is a cop-out. **T F**

6. People lose weight more quickly from exercise that is in the mid-range of exertion than they do from exercise that's in the high range of exertion. In other words, jogging is better for weight loss than sprinting. **T F**

7. Exercise has been demonstrated by research to help prevent cardiovascular disease, but its effects on other diseases have yet to be scientifically proven, regardless of what faddists may say. **T F**

8. The old feel-the-burn technique is outdated. Most exercise physiologists now say it's better to push your muscles to the brink of fatigue, then back off. **T F**

9. Primarily because of psychological factors, the more quickly you can lose weight, the better off you'll be—unless you do it so quickly that you become depleted, and harm your health. **T F**

The Answers: They're all false. Some of the questions were kind of tricky, though. Here are some explanations.

1. A 30-minute workout actually decreases hunger by producing stimulating chemicals, such as adrenaline, and by triggering the burning of body fat for energy.

2. Old wives' tale. Muscle cannot become fat. Muscles just get smaller when you discontinue exercising.

3. Spot reducing is a myth. You can tone muscles in specific areas, but it won't make the fat in those areas go away any faster than exercising the entire body does.

4. It's better to exercise for an hour straight. Muscles grow best from being exhausted, and that generally occurs during longer periods of exercise.

5. The main reason women have more body fat than men is because of their hormones, not lack of physical activity. The deck is stacked against women. Sad but true.

6. Another myth. The harder you work out, the faster you'll lose weight. But hard work often wears people out too quickly, and then they stop completely. That's how the easy-does-it myth got started.

7. Research shows that exercise helps prevent everything from cancer to Alzheimer's to minor illnesses.

8. The burn works. It just hurts, that's all.

9. Slow but sure is the way to go. Be patient. Patience pays.

The Seven Immediate Effects of Exercise

When You Work Out, This Will Happen *Today*

1. Exercise releases fat-burning hormones. The hormones thyroxin (a thyroid hormone), norepinephrine (an adrenal hormone), and testosterone (a steroid hormone) are all immediately increased by exercise. And they all radically invigorate the process of burning body fat.

Exercise changes the hormonal profiles of people with "sluggish" thyroid glands—one of the primary causes of gaining weight easily.

Exercise also helps people who tend to have slow metabolisms by stimulating the release of the adrenal hormone norepinephrine.

In addition, exercise causes increased production of the male hormone testosterone, which is critically important for building muscle mass and burning body fat. Women's bodies have testosterone—just not as much as men's bodies—and it's a key element in not only energy and muscle building, but also in enhancing sexual desire. The higher amount of testosterone among males is the primary reason they tend to be less overweight than females.

When all three of these hormones are released, they increase the efficiency and rate of the metabolism by up to 15 percent, and this lasts for several hours. This is the main reason exercise keeps burning body fat even after you stop exercising.

2. Exercise burns calories. In fact, the physical demands of the body are the only thing that burns calories. To burn off one pound of body fat, you need to burn off about 3,500 calories. Because it usually takes about one hour of moderate exercise to burn off 500 calories, a rule of thumb is that approximately one half-hour of exercise every day of the week burns off about one pound of body fat every two weeks.

By the same token, if you avoid eating about 3,500 extra calories every two weeks, or about 250 per day, you can also lose about one pound of fat every two weeks.

Therefore, if you exercise half an hour a day, plus cut your food intake by about 250 calories per day, you can lose about one pound each week.

3. Exercise decreases hunger. Sounds counterintuitive, but it's true. Exercise decreases hunger not only because it spurs production of the stimulating hormones thyroxin, norepinephrine, and testosterone, but also because it increases the levels of the stimulating neurotransmitter dopamine. These body chemicals can kill hunger even better than eating can.

These same energizing chemicals can cause insomnia, though, if you exercise just before bedtime. So try to work out in the morning.

Another way exercise kills hunger is by triggering the body to start burning body fat—instead of burning dietary calories. When that process kicks in, it can knock out your hunger for hours. In effect, you're digesting your own fat.

4. Exercise regulates insulin levels. The whole low-carb movement is based on the fact that carbohydrates (starch and sugar) cause spikes of excessive insulin production. Having these spikes of insulin leads to hunger, overeating, and excessive storage of calories as body fat. You can escape these spikes by avoiding sugar or starch-filled calories. But another great way to control insulin is with exercise. Exercise makes the cells more sensitive to insulin, which helps hold down insulin production.

Even people who don't lose weight from exercise still benefit tremendously from its effect on insulin, because it makes them less prone to diabetes, even if they're still overweight.

5. Exercise boosts mood and mental function. Exercise is practically as powerful as the best medications, such as antidepressants, for fighting depression and anxiety. This is mostly because it increases stimulating, energizing hormones, and raises the levels of the neurotransmitter dopamine. Plus, it increases endorphin levels by about 500 percent.

Improved mood, in turn, helps prevent overeating due to emotional reasons.

In addition, exercise improves cognitive function, including memory and reasoning skills. It's so beneficial that it's now considered a primary preventive measure against Alzheimer's.

6. Exercise increases muscle mass, which accelerates body-fat burning. Muscle tissue burns up to 20 percent more calories than does body fat, even when the muscles are at rest. This is one of the reasons men lose weight more easily than women: Their additional musculature is a veritable fat-burning furnace.

Women, though, can still make weight management easier by adding extra muscle.

Contrary to an old myth, this muscle will not become fat if exercise is discontinued—the size of the muscle will simply be reduced.

7. Exercise prevents disease. Exercise not only improves mood and energy levels, but also confers resistance to many diseases, including most of the deadly degenerative diseases, such as heart disease, stroke, cancer, diabetes, and Alzheimer's.

Exercise is exceptionally effective for preventing cardiovascular diseases. In general, it's even more beneficial for prevention than medication is.

It is also surprisingly effective for helping to reduce the risk of cancer. Studies show that it decreases the risk of cancer of the reproductive organs by 250 percent, breast cancer by 200 percent, and colon cancer by 67 percent.

It is also effective for helping control chronic pain (because of its effects on neurotransmitters), and even helps prevent memory-loss diseases, such as multiple minor strokes.

All of these effects begin to happen immediately. Not tomorrow. Today.

The Magic Half-Hour

When I Exercise, How Long Is Enough?

Realistically? A half-hour is enough. Less than that isn't.

All the workouts in this book are half-hour sessions, plus a little warm-up and a short cooldown. If you keep your heart rate elevated the entire thirty minutes, you will almost certainly lose weight.

What's so magical about a half-hour?

If you exercise for a half-hour, your body will burn fat. If you exercise for less than that, you probably won't.

Even if you're eating a relatively low-carb diet, all you burn is blood sugar, or glucose, for the first ten to fifteen minutes that you exercise. First, you burn the glucose that's in your bloodstream. After that, you burn the glucose that's stored in your liver and muscles.

Then comes the good part. Your body stops running on readily available blood sugar, and you shift into the extraordinary beneficial act of burning body fat.

As you begin to burn your own body fat, this fat begins to provide you with the energy you need to continue your day's activities. It's almost as if you are constantly eating. Your body is consuming its own fat for energy, in much the same way that it consumes food for energy.

The beauty of this is:

* **You're not hungry.** You have a source of sustenance.
* **You're losing weight.**

Nice one–two combination, huh?

A lot of people, however, stop exercising before they make this important transition into body-fat burning. If you make the mistake of quitting too early, guess what happens to you?

You stay hungry. In fact, you often feel famished, because you've depleted not only your bloodstream's glucose but also the glucose that's stored in your liver and muscles. But you're not burning body fat yet, so you have no source of sustenance. When this happens, you fall into that terrible condition known as hypoglycemia, or low blood sugar.

This is unfortunate, because low blood sugar feels awful. You get weak, shaky, tired, irritable, forgetful—and ravenously hungry.

The only thing worse than how hypoglycemia feels is the absolute havoc it wreaks upon your body. Every episode of hypoglycemia kills and damages cells throughout your body. In effect, hypoglycemia starves them to death.

One part of your body that is hit especially hard is your brain. The reason you feel so bad mentally and emotionally when your blood sugar gets low is because hypoglycemia starves your brain. Your brain is particularly vulnerable simply because it uses so much of your blood sugar. It uses 20 percent of all available glucose. When this glucose is depleted, brain cells are damaged and killed. In fact, you can kill as many brain cells from an episode of hypoglycemia as you can from getting drunk on alcohol.

Besides battering your brain, low blood sugar also hurts your insulin system, the part of your hormonal system that gives your cells a steady supply of the energy from blood sugar. Insulin carries your blood sugar into your cells.

When blood sugar in the cells gets too low, the cells trigger the release of more insulin, as they cry out for more sugar to be carried in to them. When this sugar arrives, it makes you feel okay for a few minutes, but pretty soon your glucose runs out again, and you feel worse than ever.

The more often hypoglycemia hits, the more vulnerable to it you become. Your body eventually trains itself to pump out big, erratic surges of insulin.

- **You begin to get hungry more easily.**
- **You gain weight much more easily, because your overactive insulin system makes you hoard calories.**
- **The fatter you get, the worse your insulin system functions.**
- **Your insulin system gradually fails, as you progress from hypoglycemia, to prediabetes, to diabetes.**

Meanwhile, you're cursing fate: I work out! I shouldn't be fat! I shouldn't have diabetes! **You can prevent this.**

One way to help prevent it is to just work out a little longer. Don't quit after the first ten or fifteen minutes, at that point when your body has burned up all its easily available blood sugar. Instead, keep exercising until you make the transition to body-fat burning. It will probably take only a few more minutes.

This transition is, in fact, the primary element of the commonly experienced "second wind" that occurs during extended exercise.

If you keep exercising until you start to burn body fat, you'll discover that just as your body trains itself to overproduce insulin, it can also train itself to make the transition to body-fat burning. The more often you make this transition, the easier it gets.

However, just feeling a lot better isn't the only thing that happens when you make this transition. The other thing that occurs when you make the transition to burning body fat is, of course, that you lose weight.

This is why you should exercise for about a half-hour, straight, without taking any appreciable breaks.

This is why I call a half-hour workout the Magic Half-Hour.

Since thirty minutes is the magic number for benefiting from exercise, all the workouts in this book are designed to take about thirty minutes, plus a short warm-up and cooldown. Probably none of them will last exactly a half-hour, though, because people do them at different paces. Therefore, when you do the workouts, make sure they last thirty minutes—by adding a little more work at the end if necessary. However, if you don't finish all the exercises in thirty minutes, it's okay to leave out a few of the exercises or reps. Of course, it's much better to go a little over the half-hour than under it. If you have the energy and time to go over, go for it.

Chapter 5

Phase Two
Your New Body

Welcome to Phase Two

You've made it. **You're past the first two weeks of my program.** You made yourself get started, and starting is always harder than continuing. Instead of inertia, you have momentum. Now it's time to take it to the next level.

Let's make this even more invigorating.

Phase Two is a bit more vigorous than Phase One, but as I mentioned earlier, it's going to feel easier because you've already built some muscle and burned some fat—even if it's not really showing yet.

By the end of this phase, though, it will show. You'll have a new body by the end of this phase. The body you're going to get in the next two weeks will be new to you, and it will be the stronger, leaner body that will empower you to soon enter the final phase, when you'll really begin to see results.

Phase Two not only introduces somewhat more active workouts, but also grapples with more refined, sophisticated concepts regarding the other three elements of fitness: (1) your mind and spirit, (2) your eating habits, and (3) your efforts to cleanse your body of toxins.

As in Phase One, we'll first cover the mind, then food, then cleansing, and finally exercise. Don't stop working out while you read all this material. Skip ahead to today's workout, and do it today, as you begin to read the rest of the Phase Two information.

Get ready for results. You're going to see your body change over the next two weeks. And so will other people.

Phase Two | **Fitness Element #1** | *Mind and Spirit*

Phase Two: Creating a New Body with Your Mind and Your Spirit

The Phase One material on the mental and spiritual elements of fitness was mostly about challenging yourself: finding your motivation, overcoming your inertia, and facing down your fears. In Phase Two, the new theme is self-exploration. Now it's time to look within, and find the inner resources that are going to change your body and change your life.

You'll examine your intent, your expectations, your inner dialogue about your body, your natural human resistance to hard work, and your own, specific fitness problems.

This will be interesting.

And remember, whatever you find in yourself: Use it.

Talk to Yourself

I hate going to a gym where they have music blasting, supposedly to pep people up. I wear earplugs.

When I work out, I want to focus on my body, and not be distracted by a disco ball and loud music. I want to be able to hear myself think. I want to be able to talk to myself, and connect to my workout.

It's important to talk to yourself as you work out, especially if you're like most people and don't have a personal trainer talking to you. Most people need to be their own personal trainer. In your case, I want you to let me be your personal trainer, even though I won't be physically present. I want you to hear my voice inside your head, urging you to work hard, have fun, and stay focused.

Along with my voice, I want you to hear your own voice. When you do talk to yourself, I want you to do it the same way that I talk to my clients—the same way I'd talk to you if I were in the room.

Just as there's a right way and a wrong way to do almost every exercise, there's a right way and a wrong way to talk to yourself during exercise.

Language has power. Dr. Dan Baker, a psychologist at Arizona's famous Canyon Ranch spa—where many of my clients go for R & R, and to work on their personal growth—says that language has the power to change lives. For a long time, Dr. Baker believed that people used language mostly just to describe the world they saw. But then he realized that as people described things, they defined them, and created what these things meant in their own lives.

In other words: We don't just describe the world we see; we see the world we describe.

As you progress in my One Body, One Life program, and begin to change your life, you'll probably notice that the kind of language you use will begin to change. As you improve yourself, you'll naturally tend to start using language that's more constructive—instead of neutral or destructive. You'll begin to shy away from overusing negative, self-defeating words like "can't" and "shouldn't" and "won't." You'll unconsciously start to describe the world around you more positively. You'll see possibilities where you used to just see problems. You'll start to describe your own actions in the active voice, instead of the passive voice.

Just as changing your life will change your language, changing your language will change your life. The way you talk to yourself helps determine how you see yourself. How you see yourself helps determine the person you are.

How should you talk to yourself? Simple: the same way you want other people to talk to you.

Let's say you're in the gym. Do you want your trainer to criticize you or make fun of you? Of course not. You want to be treated with respect. So you need to learn to treat yourself with respect.

When you're working out, you need to talk to yourself the same way I talk to all my clients—famous or unknown, rich or struggling.

How I Talk to My Clients

- **In a positive way.** They don't want me to tear them down. They want me to build them up. They want my trust, support, and enthusiasm. They want praise. And they deserve it.
- **In a compassionate way.** Compassion, of course, is more than just being positive. It's empathy. It's me knowing that what my clients are doing is hard. It's caring about their struggles. It's respect.
- **In a technically precise way.** A good trainer—even if you're your own trainer—has got to be more than just a cheerleader. A good trainer, or a self-trainer, has to know the proper techniques—as you will by the end of this book. Then, after you know them, you've got to talk yourself into doing them.

  When I'm working out, I'll be talking to myself about my pinkie finger squeezing the weight bar. I'll be talking to myself about how far I'm bringing the weight down. I'll be asking myself if my arm is flat against the pad, and if my neck is relaxed. Technique is everything. (Remember: If you're not doing it right, you're not doing it.) The best way to do it right is to talk yourself through it.

- **In a focused way.** I talk a lot about focus in this chapter, because focus is a primary element of how you use your mind during exercise. But you can't just think about focus. You've got to talk to yourself about it. Thinking can get muddy in a hurry, because it's hard to think about just one thing at a time. Other thoughts always crowd in. It's easier to focus when you talk to yourself, because the act of putting ideas into words will bring you the clarity you need.

When you talk to yourself, though, it doesn't matter if you talk out loud, or talk silently. Just the act of mentally expressing things in words is enough.

So from here on, I want you to hear my voice in your head every time you work out. And I want you to hear your own voice. You're not in this alone any longer. I'll be there. And so will your own best supporter: You!

✳ AN EXERCISE FOR YOUR SPIRIT

Here are two lists: (1) common positive self-assessments, and (2) common negative self-assessments.

Circle the three from each list that you most often say to yourself, or think to yourself. Or, make up your own most common positive and negative self-assessments.

The next time you work out, focus on not saying any of the three negatives, and saying all three of the positives.

Then, try it again, during another workout.

When you reach the point where you can do this with relative ease during a workout, challenge yourself to go an entire week without saying any of the negatives, and also saying all of the positives, each day.

During your week of Positive Self-Talk, if the negative phrases do creep into your mind, visually put a big, red X over them, and immediately replace them with a positive.

POSITIVES
- I can do this if . . .
- Listen to my breath . . .
- Engage my pinkie . . .
- The best part of . . .
- Give me five more . . .
- Now give me ten more . . .
- I'm getting stronger in . . .
- The easiest part is . . .
- I'm doing better than . . .
- Relax my . . .
- Lift with my . . .
- My body looks better . . .

NEGATIVES
- I'm too weak to . . .
- I can't . . .
- This is too hard . . .
- I'll never . . .
- I wish I were . . .
- Just get the weight up . . .
- I'm not good at . . .
- This hurts my . . .
- I'm not as good as . . .
- This isn't fun . . .
- I don't like my . . .
- I look fat when . . .

POSITIVES	NEGATIVES
• I love the feeling of . . .	• I'm too lazy to . . .
• This is fun . . .	• I'm out of energy . . .
• I'm really good at . . .	• My problem is . . .

What to Do When You Don't Feel Like Working Out

A famous actress comes in for her workout, but I can see by her darting eyes that she's distracted.

Her head's just not into exercise today. She doesn't have her game face on.

Big mistake. The body follows the mind. It's time for her to get into this, or get out of it. Time to go all out, or go home.

She has reasons for her lack of interest, of course, and they're good ones. She just lost a role she really wanted. Her boyfriend just left town to shoot on location. She—

Save your breath, my friend.

I offer her plenty of compassion—because she deserves it—but I can't give her what she really needs by just listening to her problems.

What she needs—and what you need, too—is an absolute insistence on creating a sacred space in the day devoted only to fitness. After all, you've only got one body, just as you only have one life, and that body deserves its own time, every day.

I don't give my actress a sermon about the importance of exercise. That kind of condescension is self-defeating. (Never talk to yourself like that.) Instead, I just present to her the three most logical options as follows:

An Exercise for Your Spirit
for the Times When Your Head's Just Not Into It

Option #1: Call it a day. You do have that freedom. In fact, if you don't realize you have that freedom, you'll feel like you're in Exercise Jail, and you'll eventually grow to hate your workouts.

Exercise is a choice, and choice is the foundation of freedom. If you don't accept the fact that you have power over your own choices, you'll lose your sense of controlling your own life and your own body. You'll be resentful and rebellious.

This doesn't mean, of course, that it's smart to choose every day not to exercise. If you do that, you're not exerting your free will—you're just giving in to apathy.

Option #2: Physicalize your emotions. The main reason most people don't feel like working out is because they're preoccupied with their daily problems, and weighed down with the lethargy that comes with those problems.

You can physicalize what's on your mind, and work through it—and past it. You probably physicalize your emotions all the time, without even being aware of it. For example, when you get off the phone after a difficult business call and you smack your hand on your desk, that's physicalizing your emotions. Or, if you throw your hands up into the air, that's physicalizing your emotions.

In fact, it's virtually impossible not to physicalize your emotions, because the mind and body are inseparable. The body almost always responds to what's going on in the mind, in one way or another. Too often, though, the way it responds to negative emotions is with subtle tightening and tensing. A lot of people allow this to go on all day long, until by the end of the day their necks are like coiled steel, and they feel as if they've been in a fight. They *have* been in a fight—a fight with themselves.

The classic American way to get rid of this accumulated tension at the end of the day is to drink it away during a happy hour, eat it away during dinner, or numb it away in front of the television. Or, a combination of all three.

There's a better way.

First, don't tense up. Physicalize the little stressful moments during your day as they occur, to keep your tension from adding up. Don't be afraid to smack your desk with your hand, or stomp your foot, or raise your voice a little.

Stress-release techniques don't have to be forceful movements, though. Just stretching can get rid of a lot of pent-up emotion, especially if you stretch your neck and shoulders where tension loves to live. The point is, you're human—so don't be afraid to act like it. Women, especially, hold in too much tension, because of old-fashioned ideas about acting ladylike.

You shouldn't make a scene, though, and you certainly shouldn't turn your anger or frustration against somebody else. If you do, you'll just end up with more problems than you started with. Let the people around you know you're not really losing your temper, and that you're not mad at them. If you do this, you can engage in a little bit of healthy catharsis as the day goes along, without hurting anyone's feelings, or calling undue attention to yourself.

Then, when it comes time to work out: Watch out, world! Now you can get cathartic in a big way. And it's going to feel good.

To physicalize your emotions during a workout, you should focus intently on your anger, frustration, boredom—or whatever's got you down—and then beat it up. You'll be amazed at how much better you'll feel in a shockingly short time.

Some types of exercise are better for stress release than others. The best kind, for most people, are the exercises that safely mimic fighting, such as the martial arts. A few kicks and punches are great for releasing your emotions in a healthy way.

It can also feel great to do some rugged outdoor work, such as splitting firewood, pulling up weeds, digging, or hammering. Even just jogging or running can let off a tremendous amount of steam.

When you physicalize your emotions, a funny thing will happen: You'll have more energy after you work out than you did before. It takes a lot of energy to hold in feelings.

Option #3: Create an emotional oasis. When you begin your workout, you can just drop your negative emotions. You have that power. You can check them at the door, and enter into a world that's free from your ordinary worries. Doing this is just a matter of willpower.

You probably already do this all the time, without really thinking about it. For example, you probably forget your everyday cares when you go to the movies. You just decide to let the world solve its own problems for a couple of hours, while you kick back and escape into an environment that feels like it's been created just for you.

Your workout can become your own daily oasis. It can be your free time away from your concerns about your kids, your finances, your boss, or any other nagging worries.

Achieving this experience of emotional oasis just takes a little practice. Do it a few times, and you'll see how easy it is. It's easy for a simple reason: It feels good.

The Choice Is Yours

You may be wondering, what did my client choose to do that day about her own disinterest in exercise?

She chose to physicalize her feelings. That approach was the one that most closely fit her mood that day. I had to urge her on for a short time—but, boy, did she get into it! She felt much better afterward.

And, she soon got another role that was even better than the one she'd lost. And her boyfriend returned, as boyfriends generally do.

That's how problems are: They seem like the end of the world at the time, but they hardly ever last.

You'll always have another problem—I guarantee it.

But you'll never have another body.

Phase Two | Fitness Element #2 | *Power Food*

Phase Two: Creating a New Body with Power Food

You received the basics in Phase One: counting calories and eating healthy. It's time to move on to the next step.

Let's look at some of the more complex issues: low-carb vs. low-fat, the menace of yeast overgrowth, the terrible risk you take when you allow yourself to get hungry, and weight-loss vs. weight-maintenance dieting.

These are issues you need to understand. They go beyond mere common sense, into the realm of food science.

Some of this info is going to be very good news. You'll find that eating right is by no means just a matter of willpower. It's also a matter of savvy and sophistication. Your new knowledge will be your new power.

Low-Carb? or Low-Fat?

All this confusion about the so-called "low-carb vs. low-fat" conflict is nothing more than just the media making money.

There's no conflict. There should be no confusion.

It serves the agenda of the media to make you think that there's a hot new approach to weight loss—and that everything you know is wrong. This is ridiculous. Carbs and fat are both fattening, and should be carefully limited. It's always been that way, and it will always be that way.

- Carbs (starch and sugar) are fattening mostly because they can destabilize blood-sugar levels. This creates hunger and cravings.
- Fat is fattening mostly because it's high in calories—about 250 percent higher in calories than the same volume of carbs or protein.

You'll never get thin eating too much sugar and starch.
You'll never get thin eating too much fat.

To get thin, eat a lean-protein diet that's rich in nutrients and low in fat and carbs. It's really that simple.

WHEN YOU READ FOOD LABELS, LOOK FOR THIS:

Serving size:	Be aware that that little candy bar that doesn't seem to have many calories might be two servings, or even three.
Calories:	This is key. Look at calories first.
Fat:	Pay close attention to fat! Here are reasonable levels per serving.
Saturated fat:	0 to 0.5 g. Look out for saturated fats! They're terrible.
Trans fat:	Absolutely 0 g. Avoid it completely.

Polyunsaturated fat:	Up to 5 g is acceptable.
Monusaturated fat:	Up to 5 g is acceptable.
Cholesterol:	Up to 20 g is acceptable.
Sodium:	If it's more than 200 mg, avoid it.
Dietary fiber:	The more, the better.
Expiration date:	This is important. Eating fresh food really makes a difference.

You Don't Get Thin from Being Hungry— You Get Thin from Being Full

You should never be hungry. Ever. Hunger is nothing more than a disease symptom.

The disease is hypoglycemia, or low blood sugar. (Technically, hypoglycemia is classified as a "condition," rather than a disease, but that's just a matter of medical jargon. The point is, hunger isn't healthy.)

Here are the symptoms most people associate with hunger:

- A strong urge to eat—more than mere desire: a "need to feed" response.
- Feelings of physical weakness or fatigue.
- Difficulty concentrating for extended periods.
- Moderate irritability, or depression.

These are all symptoms of hypoglycemia. And every time you experience them, your body is deteriorating.

- Muscle cells are dying.
- Brain cells are dying.
- Organ cells are dying.
- Your endocrine glands are being exhausted by having to pump out extra adrenal hormones and insulin.
- You're moving closer to diabetes.
- You're moving closer to being overweight or obese.

This constellation of decline gets a little worse each additional time you get hungry. It all adds up, over time. It creates a cascade of deterioration.

To be healthy, slim, and fit, you must keep your blood-sugar levels stable. That means no more getting hungry.

The good news: Keeping your blood-sugar levels stabilized feels better than letting them become unstable. Nobody likes being hungry. Hunger hurts.

How Not to Be Hungry

Think of your blood sugar as a fire that must continually be fed. Feed it before the fire goes out. Don't wait to get hungry before you eat. Eat just before you get hungry. You know when you're going to get hungry: about two to four hours after the last time you ate, depending on how active you are. Eat by the clock, not by the sound of your stomach growling.

The simplest way to do this is just to eat three good meals and three good snacks every day. "Good" means healthy food—high-protein, high-fiber food that will burn slowly and stick to your ribs. Keep the carbs low, because they'll burn too fast, spike up your insulin, and then drop you like a bad habit.

Eating three good meals and three good snacks every day will kill your hunger forever.

If you start to get hungry anyway, eat. Just eat healthy food. Not soda pop. Not a candy bar. (That also means: Not a diet shake. And not a nutrition bar.) Good, wholesome food.

The only time you should ever get hungry is if you're out on a hike, or out on a boat, and can't find anything to eat. Other than that, you should never be hungry.

It's just not how fit people live.

✳ AN EXERCISE IN NUTRITION
An exercise I often do with clients is to have them set their watch or an alarm clock to go off every three hours. When it rings, they have to eat. It might just be a light snack of ten raw almonds, but they have to put something in their mouth. Obviously, this keeps them from being hungry, and it stops them from overeating. It's an exercise in consistency, satiety, and good habits. Try it! You'll love never being hungry. You'll love the energy. And you'll really love the fact that you'll lose weight.

Build Your Body's Response to Exercise

People sometimes tell me that no matter how hard they work out, their bodies just don't seem to respond. They exercise regularly but still don't lose weight.

These people often blame the aging process. They complain that they're getting older, and their metabolisms are slowing down.

That's generally not the real problem. Metabolic slowdown is mostly a myth. The rate of human metabolism decreases by only about 1 percent every decade.

Furthermore, many of the people who say that they don't lose weight from exercise aren't even old. They're in their twenties or early thirties.

The real reason for this lack of weight loss from exercise—among both young people and older people—is often because these people have too much stored blood sugar in their systems.

When you have too much stored blood sugar, you tend to just burn blood sugar when you exercise, and not body fat. You can work out hard, but still be unable to achieve much weight loss.

Your body stores blood sugar in two ways. Some is stored right in the bloodstream. Other blood sugar is stored in the liver and muscles. The blood sugar that's stored in the liver and muscles is called glycogen.

Your body burns practically all of this blood sugar before it even starts to burn body fat.

Athletes are aware of this principle, and they try to use it to their advantage. They often try to build up their levels of glycogen before they compete in marathons, or other endurance events. They know that when they start running, they'll burn up all the blood sugar in their bloodstream within a matter of minutes, and will then begin to burn the glycogen in their liver and muscles. Therefore, they want to have as much glycogen as possible.

Eventually their bodies will burn up most or all of their glycogen. Then their bodies will begin to burn body fat for energy.

However, burning body fat for energy isn't quite as efficient as burning pure blood sugar. It's almost as efficient, but nothing quite compares to oxidizing pure sugar for quick energy. This drop in efficiency isn't really noticeable to the average person during the course of a normal day, or even a vigorous workout, but it can be noticeable to an athlete in the midst of a long, grueling, competitive event.

Therefore, athletes in long races usually try to postpone this shift to body-fat burning.

There's only one way to do that: by increasing the amount of blood sugar that's stored in the liver and muscles. And there's only one way to increase this storage: by eating high amounts of carbohydrates—because carbs are converted almost instantly into blood sugar, and the excess is quickly stored away. This well-known strategy is called carbo-loading.

When endurance athletes carbo-load before a big event, they can postpone their shift to body-fat burning by up to two hours, or sometimes even longer.

Carbo-loading is a clever strategy—but only for endurance athletes competing in big events. For you, it's a disaster.

On a day-to-day basis, you should try to do the exact opposite of carbo-loading, in order to get your body to shift to the burning of body fat as quickly as possible during your workout.

The opposite of carbo-loading, of course, is limiting your intake of carbs. If you limit carbs, you will naturally reduce your glucose levels in your bloodstream, and the glycogen in your liver and muscles. You'll then start burning body fat as quickly as possible when you exercise.

This quick shift to body-fat burning will make a huge difference in your body's responsiveness to exercise. Instead of just burning blood sugar when you exercise, you'll burn body fat. Instead of exercising for thirty minutes and seeing no discernible results, you'll exercise for thirty minutes and see the difference. You will, in fact, begin to respond to exercise in the same effective, efficient way that thin people seem to respond to it.

Phase Two | Fitness Element #3 | *Cleansing*

Phase Two: Creating a New Body with Cleansing

In Phase One, I introduced the idea that you just can't get fit if your body is burdened with toxins. They can sap your energy, change your mood, and ruin the delicate balance of your metabolism.

Now we get even more proactive. In this phase, you do a one-day Weekend Cleanse. You're going to crack down on toxins—with a comprehensive program designed to drive them out of your system.

What's Eating You?

Parasites may have invaded your body, and may still be living within your gastrointestinal tract, or in other tissues. This is much more common than most people realize, and it can create a terrible drain on your energy and health.

Everybody knows that when you travel to a foreign country—particularly a Third World country—you run a risk of contracting a parasite from the local water. Many people, however, even contract miniscule parasites in America from drinking the local water, when they travel from one city to another.

What most people don't realize is that parasites are abundant even within our own immediate, home environments, and frequently cause health problems that are commonly misdiagnosed as the flu, chronic fatigue, or other illnesses. Very often, even people with very healthy lifestyles suffer from extended low energy, malaise, or gastrointestinal distress, without knowing that the problem isn't a virus, a bacteria, irritable bowel syndrome, or stress—it's a parasite. These debilitating symptoms can have a catastrophic impact upon fitness.

Here are some of the places parasites come from:

- **Your family pet.** Especially if you nuzzle your pet's face a lot. Pets are notorious carriers of parasites.
- **Improperly cooked foods.** Pork is often a culprit (causing trichinosis), but other meats can also harbor parasites. Even fruits and vegetables can have them. And

sushi can be a source, too, if it's undercooked (ha ha). (Hint: Eat sushi with wasabi and pickled ginger, which help kill parasites.)

- **Tap water.** It doesn't have to be from a Third World country. Many American cities have impure water. That's why bottled water is now so popular.
- **Restaurants.** The most likely to spread parasites are mom-and-pop diners and delis that don't have strict food-handling policies.

These sources of parasites harbor:

- **Single-cell parasites.** These parasites include the very common giardia. This is a microscopic, water-borne parasite often found in swimming pools, lakes, hot tubs, and bathrooms. Another common single-cell parasite is *Toxoplasma gondii*, which is believed to be present in small quantities in up to one-fourth of the American population. A common source of toxoplasma is cat litter.
- **Flukes.** These tiny parasites are often found in animals. They can also be transferred to people from undercooked fish and crabs, and from leafy vegetables, including watercress.
- **Roundworms and tapeworms.** They're present in a relatively large percentage of America's pets (up to 25 percent of cats), and can be spread to people who play with pets. An estimated 25 percent of the world's population has roundworms.

If any of these parasites are in your system, you may have these symptoms: fatigue, bloating, gas, constipation, diarrhea, skin rash, lassitude, or nausea.

YOUR TO-DO LIST

For centuries, people have been successfully eliminating parasites with noninvasive herbal therapies. It's easy, quick, painless, and effective.

These days, there are also appropriate pharmaceutical medications for parasites, including praziquantel (for flukes and tapeworms), mebendazole (for roundworms), and metronidazole (for giardiasis). However, because it's hard to definitely determine the presence of parasites, it is probably more appropriate for most people to employ the herbal therapies. They are far less likely to cause side effects, and they're usually quite effective. The best natural remedies are:

Immune Elixir. It's the general immune tonic that I recommend in the Phase Three section on supplements. It has an array of herbs that kill parasites.

Garlic. It contains the active antipathogen constituent called allicin. It's particularly effective against giardia, the swimming-pool parasite. Take as directed on the bottle.

Goldenseal. It has traditionally been used for conditions that affect the mucous membranes, which tend to harbor fungi, bacteria, and parasites. Take as directed.

Other remedies. Black walnut, available at some health-food stores, may help. So might Chinese wormwood. Another home remedy is to eat approximately one-third of a cup of un-cooked short-grain rice, chewing carefully to dissolve it, with no other foods. This helps to gather and expel toxic material in the digestive tract.

Like other methods of detoxification, attempting to kill parasites may not have a notice-able effect upon you—or it might change your whole life. It's certainly worth eating some garlic to find out!

Three Great Detoxifiers

These Three Supplements Are of Special Value

Garlic. Garlic has the power to selectively bind with, or chelate, heavy metals—particularly lead and mercury. It can increase bowel excretion of mercury by 400 percent. Recommended daily dosage: 750–1,500 mg.

Selenium. It binds with and deactivates mercury, and is one of the strongest antioxidants. Recommended daily dosage: 100–300 mg.

Vitamin C. It chelates numerous toxins and heavy metals, including carbon monoxide, pesti-cides, arsenic, cadmium, chromium, chlorine, aluminum, and fluoride. Recommended daily dosage: up to a maximum of 3–4 g.

✺ AN EXERCISE IN CLEANSING

Cleansing can involve not only the body, but also the mind. There is such a thing as "toxic thoughts." The word we usually use for these toxic thoughts is "stress." Stress kills. It constricts arteries, it burns the brain with neurohormones, and it drastically impairs immunity. It can even change your whole perspective on life.

There are a hundred ways to bust stress and free yourself from toxic thoughts—but here's one you may not have considered. Pick an evening and try to remain in the calming cocoon of silence for the rest of the night. If you need to communicate, write it down. You'll find that after a while, you'll naturally slip past the boundaries of verbal communication, and be able to easily communicate nonverbally. You move into a different plane of communication and connecting.

At first, your mind will be full of inner dialogue—the surface chatter that clutters our lives. Soon, all this just dissolves.

The payoff is peace. Peace within your family. Peace within yourself.

Once you get into it, you may even choose to go an entire weekend day without talking.

Silence is the language of healing.

The Phase Two Weekend Cleanse: A Powerful Technique for Rejuvenation

The Weekend Cleanse is a fantastic regimen of detoxification that may help you feel better than you have in years, if you suffer from a significant accumulation of toxins. It is specifically designed to help expel toxins that are lodged in cells, and in the organs of elimination.

My Weekend Cleanse was designed, in part, by Robert Abbatiello, N.D., L.Ac., who has worked on cleansing programs for many years. Dr. Abbatiello has made a science out of ridding the body of toxins.

Most of my clients really enjoy the Weekend Cleanse, because of the sense of energy and renewal it sparks. My rock-star client Pink is a big fan of cleansing, and has even done it on tour.

In Phase Two, you should do the Weekend Cleanse for one day. It may be on either Saturday or Sunday, and it should be done on the first and second week of the phase.

In Phase Three, you do the Weekend Cleanse one more time, but you do it for both days of the weekend. That will give you an even greater lift.

The only thing that is at all challenging about the Weekend Cleanse is drinking a nutritional drink, called the Liver Flush, that doesn't taste very good to most people. Some people like it, but the majority just tolerate it, as one does any other kind of medicinal drink that's designed to help your health, instead of please your palate.

Here's how you do the Weekend Cleanse:

Upon Rising: Mix your two nutritional, cleansing drinks. The purpose of both is to stimulate the function of your liver and kidneys, your body's two primary organs of detoxification. The liver and kidneys can easily become congested with toxins, and this can create a back-up of toxins in your bloodstream, and in cells throughout your body. This back-up of toxins can make you feel sluggish and irritable, and it can go on for weeks or even months. Some people, in fact, live in an almost constant state of excess toxicity, and it profoundly depresses their mental and physical functions.

The first nutritional drink you prepare is called the Master Cleanser.

The Master Cleanser

Juice of 1 lemon

32 ounces spring water

1 1/2 tablespoons maple syrup or honey

1 pinch ground clove, or 1/2 teaspoon whole clove

(If you prefer, you can substitute 2–3 teaspoons of xylitol

for the syrup or honey.)

Blend the ingredients for 20–40 seconds. If desired, you may strain it.

Then you prepare the Liver Flush.

The Liver Flush

1 peeled lemon

1 peeled orange

1 ounce olive oil

3 sprigs parsley

1 1" piece of fresh ginger root

1 pinch of: ginger, cayenne, pepper, and ground clove

Blend lemon, orange, parsley, and ginger with one cup of water. Strain the pulp, return liquid to blender, add remaining ingredients. Blend again. If you prefer, you may substitute cilantro for the parsley. You may also add a teaspoon of bee pollen, if desired. After you have tried the Liver Flush once or twice, you may amplify its effects by doubling the amount of garlic, pepper, olive oil, or a bigger piece of ginger.

When both drinks are prepared:

- Drink the entire Liver Flush.
- Then drink 8 ounces of the Master Cleanser.
- Take 1,000 mg of vitamin C.
- Take 100 mg of magnesium.

This is your breakfast. Sip the rest of the Master Cleanser throughout the day.

Midmorning snack: Five to ten raw almonds, and half an apple or pear.

Thirty minutes before lunch: Drink eight ounces of fresh juice prepared with a juicer—at least 80 percent of it should be vegetable juice, and 20 percent should be fruit juice. Take another 1,000 mg of vitamin C and 100 mg of magnesium. See www.onebodyonelife.com for some great juice recipes.

Lunch: Have a big vegetable salad, with dark greens only—no red peppers or tomatoes—and four ounces of fish or chicken. For dressing, combine lemon juice and olive oil (or diluted sesame tahini, or hummus).

Afternoon snack: Five to ten raw almonds, and half of an apple or pear. Or you may have five to ten almonds, and one cup of sliced carrots, cucumber, or celery.

Thirty minutes before dinner: Drink eight more ounces of juice—80 percent vegetable, 20 percent fruit. Take one more round of supplements: 1,000 mg of vitamin C and 100 mg of magnesium. If you normally take a multivitamin, take it now.

Dinner: Eat another big vegetable salad, with dark greens only. No red peppers or tomatoes. Use the same salad dressing that you had at lunch, and add some olive oil to the potato. If you're still hungry, prepare another fresh juice, and have five to ten more almonds.

That's it. You're done.

If you have weekend plans, bring your special food and drink with you.

If your resolve is fading, use your mantra to reinvigorate your willpower. Once you experience the Weekend Cleanse, you'll realize how important it is.

Phase Two | **Fitness Element #4** | *Exercise*

Phase Two: Creating a New Body with Exercise

By the second phase of this program, you've probably begun to notice patterns in how your body responds to excercise both during and after workouts.

As you use this program to build your new body and life, you will develop a sharper sense of what your body needs and wants. As you listen to your body, you will make decisions about how to get the most out of the time you spend exercising.

The following section gets more specific about how to maximize the benefit of your workouts, and provides insights that will propel you through this important period.

As you increase your understanding of your exercise program, you will gain a better insight into what your body craves. The new body you find in Phase Two will be a catalyst for the new life you create in Phase Three and beyond.

The Myth of Spot Reducing

Where do crazy ideas like spot reducing come from? I've got a guess: They come from people who are more interested in separating you from your money than from your fat.

People want to believe that a special diet or a special exercise can selectively whittle fat off certain problem areas, such as the abdomen or the butt. Therefore, entrepreneurs exploit this desire by creating products that supposedly create weight loss in specific areas. The whole concept is nonsense.

Yes, you can build the muscles in any given area of your body. But building those muscles does not target the fat that is near those muscles.

- Doing abdominal crunches builds abdominal muscles—but it does not specifically reduce abdominal fat.
- Doing exercises for the hips and thighs builds muscles in the hips and thighs—but it does not selectively target fat in the hips and thighs.

The only way to lose fat is to lose it all over the body.

As a rule, when you lose body fat, you will first lose belly fat. Belly fat is more biologically active than lower-body fat, and generally comes off first. But belly fat will come off first regardless of what specific types of exercises you are doing. It will come off first from walking, or from doing crunches, or from lifting weights, or doing Pilates, or swimming.

The only way to lose body fat is by burning its stored calories for energy, after you've already burned the stored calories from the glucose in your bloodstream, and the glycogen in your liver and muscles. And when this body fat is oxidized for its calories, it is oxidized throughout the body (even though belly fat usually gets a little head start).

If people really could control the specific areas of their fat loss, most men would probably choose to leave some fat in their biceps, where it would look like muscle, and many women would probably choose to leave some extra fat in their breasts, in order to look more voluptuous. But have you ever been able to do this? Of course not. It's impossible—no matter how many phony ads may tell you otherwise.

Obviously, exercise can make specific areas of the body look better, by improving the muscle tone in those areas.

But if you want to lose fat—and not just gain muscle—you can usually do it more efficiently by doing generalized exercises that work the whole body. Exercises focused on very specific areas, such as the abs, exhaust these specific muscles quickly, and this fatigue tends to decrease the length of the overall workout.

Most people aren't really very interested in having strong abdominal muscles. What they really want is a thin abdomen.

There's a difference!

Of course, when your body does become thin enough for you to see your abdominal muscles, then you might want to build those muscles, to look even better.

Overcoming Inflammation

A Strategy for Preventing Mild Exercise Burnout

Not all cases of exercise burnout are characterized by dramatic, flaming crashes, when you feel like you just can't move another muscle. Much more commonly, exercise burnout just creeps up on you. You gradually begin to notice that after you work out, you feel sort of lethargic and depleted. You might feel as if you want to take a little nap, or kick back for the rest of the day. This feeling should not occur. It's not the normal reaction to an energetic workout. The normal, healthy reaction to exercise is that you have more energy *after* you work out than you did before you started. The only time it's normal to feel depleted after a workout is if you do something unusually difficult or highly strenuous.

If this type of depletion from an average workout is happening to you on a regular basis, it may be that you're suffering from a mild, widespread inflammatory reaction to exercise.

Doctors have only recently begun to realize how common the inflammatory response is, and how harmful it can be. They now believe it is a very frequent contributor to cardiovascular disease, many forms of cancer (particularly lung, breast, and prostate cancer), diabetes, arthritis, asthma, Alzheimer's, gastrointestinal disorders, and other diseases.

The reason inflammation contributes to so many different conditions is because it's a wide-ranging, systemic reaction to a huge variety of different problems—everything from bee stings to food allergies. Inflammation is basically the body's attempt to flood distressed areas with extra blood and lymphatic fluid in order to bring in healing nutrients and immune factors, and to wash away harmful substances. When a sprained ankle swells, stiffens, and becomes red, that's inflammation. When your eyes and nose are puffy and congested from hay fever, that's inflammation. When your gums bleed, that's inflammation. And there are many inflammatory reactions deep inside our bodies—and in our major organs—that we don't even notice. For example, blood vessels often become inflamed, contributing to cardiovascular disease, without any apparent symptoms.

Inflammation is a healing action. But when it becomes chronic, due to the same factor occurring again and again, it damages and kills cells.

Exercise frequently causes mild inflammation. It does it by straining and stressing muscles, and causing microscopic tears in muscle fibers. It's almost impossible to avoid at least a slight degree of inflammation in your muscles every time you work out. The sore muscles you sometimes get from exercise are primarily due to the buildup of lactic acid in them, but another reason they hurt is because of the inflammatory response.

However, soreness isn't the only sign of inflammation that's caused by exercise. A lesser degree of widespread inflammation can cause a generalized feeling of fatigue, lassitude, and lethargy, without resulting in pain. This kind of inflammation makes you feel "blah" after you work out.

This effect was demonstrated in a recent study at Emory University. People who exercised vigorously were noted to have minor muscle stresses and strains, which triggered widespread, low-level inflammation, and drained their vitality. However, when they were given aspirin after their workouts, it helped to protect their muscle cells from inflammatory stress, and they recovered from fatigue faster, and felt better.

If you commonly feel wiped out after moderate workouts, you should try to fight your inflammation. And even if you don't have any noticeable problems, it still makes sense to fight inflammation, because of its proven association with so many serious illnesses.

How to Fight Inflammation

The easy way is with aspirin. This is probably also the most powerful way.

Most people take aspirin for pain, but aspirin does more than block pain. It also reduces inflammation. Pain and inflammation are often related, but they're not the same thing. You can have inflammation without pain, and you can have pain without inflammation. Millions of people who experience no pain at all still take a small dosage of aspirin every day. They do it specifically to reduce inflammation.

Most of these people take aspirin because they know it helps prevent cardiovascular disease. For a long time, it was believed that aspirin helped prevent cardiovascular disease simply because it thins the blood, but it now appears that thinning the blood with aspirin actually may be less important for preventing cardiovascular disease than for reducing inflammation.

Because aspirin is so good at preventing heart disease, almost all doctors now advise heart patients to take an aspirin every day. A 2005 study, however, showed that aspirin helped prevent strokes among women, but didn't help prevent heart attacks among women unless they were sixty-five or older. At sixty-five, it reduced heart attacks by 25 percent. This may be because women tend to suffer heart attacks later in life than men do. The same study, though, showed that aspirin helped prevent heart attacks and strokes for men even as young as age forty-five.

Other people now take aspirin every day not just for the cardiovascular benefits, but also for its help in preventing the wide array of other common diseases that are associated with inflammation.

Ironically, aspirin appears to be emerging as the wonder drug of preventive medicine. It's apparently more beneficial for disease prevention than vitamin C, omega-3 oil, echinacea, or any of the other most popular nutrients, herbs, or formulas.

Besides aspirin, there is only one other common, over-the-counter anti-inflammatory drug: ibuprofen. Ibuprofen may someday emerge as aspirin's equal, but currently there are some doubts about its efficacy for disease prevention. A 2003 study that was reported in the medical journal *The Lancet* showed that when people took both aspirin and ibuprofen on a regular basis, the ibuprofen appeared to block the disease-preventive benefits of aspirin.

However, it's quite possible that the problem was just taking both drugs together. Further research might one day indicate that ibuprofen, when used alone, is just as helpful for disease prevention as aspirin alone. For example, another study, supported by the American Cancer Society, indicated that daily use of ibuprofen alone reduced risk of breast cancer by 20 percent.

Currently, it's impossible to know if ibuprofen will eventually prove to be as effective as aspirin for disease prevention. Therefore, it probably makes the most common sense to stick with aspirin.

One over-the-counter drug you shouldn't take for anti-inflammation, though, is acetaminophen, which is in formulas such as Tylenol. It has no anti-inflammatory effects. It's just a painkiller. (It is, however, generally considered a somewhat more powerful painkiller than either aspirin or ibuprofen.)

There are also powerful prescription anti-inflammatories—the COX-2 inhibitors, such as Celebrex. This class of drugs, though, has come under intense scrutiny due to severe side effects. At this time, it appears that these drugs are not appropriate for long-term disease prevention. They are primarily appropriate only for people with severe arthritis, or other acute inflammatory diseases.

You should be aware, though, that even innocent little aspirin can also have terrible side effects, if you take too much. The most common is gastrointestinal bleeding. Every year, people die from this. Usually, these are people with severe chronic pain, who are taking excessive dosages. Even so, you should monitor your consumption carefully. You probably should not take more than one aspirin per day, and should discontinue that immediately if you have any signs at all of gastrointestinal distress. Many doctors recommend taking even less than that. They often recommend taking a daily baby aspirin, which is only one-fourth as strong as a regular aspirin.

As with any other medication, you should talk with your doctor before beginning a regular program of aspirin use.

There are other nondrug anti-inflammatory agents, however, that appear to be risk free. These anti-inflammatories are healthy nutrients that also have numerous other benefits. You can find them at any health-food store, and many supermarkets.

YOUR TO-DO LIST

TAKE THE BIG THREE ANTI-INFLAMMATORY NUTRIENTS

- Omega-3 fish oils
- GLA (or gamma-linoleic acid, an omega-6 oil found in plants)
- Antioxidant vitamins, such as C and E

These are the best anti-inflammatory nutrients, but other nutrients can also be helpful.

TAKE SECOND-TIER ANTI-INFLAMMATORIES

- Olive oil
- B-complex vitamins
- Pycnogenol
- The amino acid glutathione
- Beta-carotene
- MSM (methylsulfonylmethane)
- The herb turmeric
- Green tea
- Garlic
- Ginger

There are also nutrients you shouldn't eat, because they contribute to the chemical process of inflammation.

AVOID THESE

- Hydrogenated fats and oils, such as margarine (Eat butter—it's a little more fattening than margarine, but much better for you.)
- Alcohol
- Sugar
- Refined starchy foods
- Saturated fats

Your normal daily diet can also help reduce inflammation. The best diet for fighting inflammation is also the same all-around diet I recommend throughout this book.

Chapter 6

Phase Three
Your New Life

Welcome to Phase Three

You rose to the challenge of change in Phase One. You changed your body in Phase Two. Now for the hard part: locking in these changes, by changing your life.

Nothing will last if you don't change your life.

But don't feel daunted, because that process has already begun. You couldn't have achieved what you already have without at least beginning to reinvent your life.

Think about it. Are you the same person you were four weeks ago? Does your mind feel the same? Your body? Do you look the same?

I doubt it. If you've stuck with my program this far, I'm certain that you have already made a commitment to yourself to lead a different kind of life, and have already started living that life. You could not have achieved what you already have without making that commitment and that change.

Keep it up. Think process, not product. Celebrate your journey, and forget about your destination.

Your journey is your new life. It is a life of movement, action, awareness, discovery, and effort without end. It's not a life for the lazy. It's the life of a traveler—the life of someone on a quest.

In this final phase, you have to continue to challenge yourself, as you did in Phase One.

And you have to continue to discover yourself, as you did in Phase Two. But now, to fully change your life—and to love that change—you must do more. Now you must do the hardest task of all.

You must accept yourself—and each moment, as it arrives—with the same love that you give to those you hold most dear.

That is the ultimate life change.

That, and only that, will empower you to live the kind of life that will lock in your fitness forever.

You can do this. You only have a little farther to go.

So begin again—as if you are beginning for the first time.

Phase Three | Fitness Element #1 | *Mind and Spirit*

Phase Three: Creating a New Life with Your Mind and Spirit

You've been very practical thus far, dealing with issues like motivation, expectation, and focus. Now it's time to get even more ambitious. The theme of Phase Three is learning to go beyond the mundane, day-to-day mental aspects of fitness, and delve into areas that are harder to describe.

For example, we will travel beyond focus, into the realm of the all-knowing unconscious, or "mindless mind." Your mindless mind has always known the secrets of fitness.

And let's try to perceive exercise as a form of meditation—because it is (or can be).

Finally, it's time to talk about how to project the new fitness you've forged, because fitness that is hidden—by bad posture, or by self-defeating style—is fitness that will eventually fade.

Remember: This is the mindset that you will be carrying into the rest of your life. Make sure you get it right. Act as if your life depends upon it.

Beyond Focus: The Mindless Mind

You've mastered focus. You're working out. You're doing stomach work. You're focusing on your breath. You're focusing on keeping your stomach tucked in. You're focusing on keeping your back relaxed. You want to do thirty reps, so you're focusing on the number thirty—you're visualizing it. You're checking in with your abs, to see if you can push things further.

Then, suddenly—out of nowhere, without even consciously trying—you become so focused, so connected to your body, that you are aware of virtually nothing except your stomach. You're living in your stomach. You are your stomach.

YOU GET IT!

At this point, you no longer need to focus. Your whole being is so wrapped up in your focus that it becomes unnecessary to think about it.

You have tapped into the power of the mindless mind. You are "thinking" with your body. This is a form of zen. I call it heart and soul training.

Your mind gets you into the "room" of heart and soul training, and then your mindless mind—your connection with your body—keeps you in the room.

Don't ever try to take a shortcut to the mindless mind of heart and soul training, however. There is no shortcut.

There is only one path to the mindless mind. The path of focus.

YOUR TO-DO LIST

This is a three-step process.

1. Try meditation. Even if you've never meditated, give it a shot. Just find a quiet place and turn off your thoughts. When they intrude, just let them go, and return to your peaceful state of nonthinking.
2. Physicalize your meditation. Do a form of exercise that is naturally relaxing and peaceful, such as a walk outside. Shut your thoughts off by focusing on the sensual, visceral elements around you: the sun, the wind, the grass, the birds.
3. Bring your meditative state to your workout. Try to do one of your daily workout routines in the meditative state. Whether it's Strength Training Day or Martial Arts Day, find a way to let your mindless mind lead the way.

The Power of Projection

All superstars have one thing in common: They know how to project themselves. They have so much personality, and put it across so well, that you just can't help but be impressed by them.

When I say "stars," I'm not talking just about actors. There are star businesspeople, star politicians, star news reporters—and star work-at-home moms. It's not the spotlight that makes the star.

Even though not all stars are famous, they all have tremendous influence within their own spheres, and are regarded by their peers with a certain degree of awe.

For example, my close friend Kevin Huvane, a partner in Hollywood's prestigious Creative Artists Agency, has as much star power as any actor in Hollywood. He's a star agent, not solely because of his brains and classiness, but also because he's mastered the power of projection. When Kevin Huvane has something to say, people listen. They don't listen just because he's got clout. They listen because he has presence.

This is also the case for my personal training client Ron Meyer, the ultrasuccessful COO of Universal Studios. You cannot be in the same room as Ron Meyer without feeling the force of his persona. He quietly radiates star power.

The same can be said of you, too, if you put some effort into it.

It's important that you learn the power of projection, because it's an integral part of fitness. It is the element of fitness that makes your mental, spiritual, and physical fitness evident to others, and even to yourself. There's just not much point in developing this fitness if you're going to hide it from the world, and from yourself. You've got to own it.

This is not a matter of simple vanity—it's a matter of self-respect. You can't command the respect of others if you don't respect yourself—and you can't fully respect yourself if you can't earn the respect of others.

You gain respect mostly by what you do. But here is a fact of life: You also gain it by how you act.

You can do great things, and be a great person, but if you act like a mousy little schlub, that's how people are going to treat you. After they treat you like that for a couple of decades, that's how you'll treat yourself. Ultimately, that's how you'll be.

Don't subvert the hard work of getting strong by acting weak. Learn to project.

The power of projection is not rocket science. Here are the basics:

Posture. Your mom was right—when you slump, people will show less respect for you. When you stand tall, you command respect. Height's not the issue; there are many leading men in Hollywood who are far smaller than they seem on-screen. They just don't "play" small.

Carriage. Carriage is your posture in motion—it's how you carry yourself. The biggest mistake most people make in how they carry themselves is that they put no effort into being graceful. Grace is worth its weight in gold. It's intrinsically attractive. But too many people march around like wooden soldiers. You can hear them coming from two rooms away. Guess how people perceive them: as stiff.

Another mistake of carriage is moving tentatively and apprehensively. When you learn to move as if you mean it, people will treat you as if you're strong, and it will amplify the strength you already have.

Eye contact is another aspect of carriage. If your eyes dart away from the person you're with, it detracts terribly from your projection of confidence and warmth. Ever see a shifty-eyed leading man, or leading lady?

Tone. Your voice is a window to your inner self. If you're a woman who has gained strength by building a relationship with your self, you don't want to betray that strength by using a weak, little-girl voice. If you do, the world will treat you like a little girl.

Similarly, if you're a stoic guy who's finally learned some sensitivity by going inside yourself, you don't want to scare people away with a monotone delivery.

Listen to how the stars use their voices. They use them like musical instruments, to convey every bit of the strength and sensitivity that they have.

Attitude. Projecting a positive image starts with projecting a positive attitude. I don't mean putting on a generic, happy-face facade. I hate facades. I mean putting the best parts of your personality out where people can see them.

If you're a cockeyed optimist, let it shine through. If one of your best traits is compassion, don't settle for just feeling it: Show it. If you're naturally courageous, let people know it.

Of course, we've also all got our dark sides—but save that side for your therapist. If you wear it on your sleeve, people won't get past it, and you'll get typecast into a role that's just a small part of you, and not the real you.

Style. Nobody knows style like the stars, and I'd like to think some of their style savvy has rubbed off on me. That doesn't mean I wear Prada every time I walk down Melrose Avenue. Style has shockingly little to do with designer labels or money. A guy like Brad Pitt can come to the gym in torn Levi's and a T-shirt, but it'll be the coolest Levi's and T-shirt you've ever seen, because it will fit his mood and his environment at that moment with immaculate precision.

Style is all about personalizing. It's about you looking like you. Fitness is relationship with self—and style is revealing that relationship. This applies not just to clothes, but also to things like hair, makeup, accessories—even the car you drive. If it's you, you'll look great, and if it's you trying to look like somebody else, you'll look like you're on your way to a costume party.

✳ AN EXERCISE FOR YOUR SPIRIT:
STAY IN CHARACTER
Pick an afternoon, or an evening—maybe a dinner date—and focus on your power of projection. Put it all together: your posture, your carriage, your tone, your attitude, and your style. Commit to the character you create.

You might find that this character is closer to the real you than you realized. Or it might open up great traits that you didn't know were there. Have fun with it! Don't come from ego. Come from courage. And don't feel surprised if you feel a little uncomfortable playing the role of this great character you're creating. That's a natural part of change and growth. Fake it 'til you make it!

A Short Story about Being Perfect:
You're not.
Epilogue:
And you never will be.
The End.

The Moral of the Story

There's nothing wrong with trying to do things perfectly. Here's why:

- When you try to do a good job, you end up doing a fair job.
- When you try to do a perfect job, you end up doing a good job.

It's fine to aspire to perfection. Keeps you hustling. But does this mean you should expect perfection? Or demand it? Only if you're out of your mind.

It's simply impossible to do things perfectly, and it's absolutely certain that you, yourself, will never be perfect. There will always be room for improvement.

Good is good enough.

Good, in fact, is great!

Don't be a perfectionist. Be a "goodist."

Expecting perfection is a mind game that's played by people who know they'll never be satisfied with themselves, no matter how good they may become.

In the end, perfectionism is just a crutch used by insecure people.

Own Your Life

To be fit, you have to own your life. You have to take personal responsibility for your actions, and work hard at controlling your own destiny.

This isn't easy. It takes courage and discipline. But there are ways to make it easier.

One of the best ways to feel as if you own your life is to keep a written record of it.

This record, over time, will help you to stay connected to your life, and when you're really connected, you're better able to own it, and control it.

If you don't keep a record of your life, it becomes harder to stay intimately connected to it, because forgetfulness can rob you of many things that you've experienced. After a while, it can almost feel as if parts of your life never even happened.

Back in the old days, many people kept track of their daily lives by keeping diaries. These days, some people keep online journals.

But both of these systems are cumbersome. Writing is hard work. Also, diaries and journals often reveal things we'd rather keep completely private. That's why old-fashioned diaries had locks.

Here's a much more practical way to create a log of your life: Keep a calendar. Just take a regular kitchen calendar, the kind with a square for each day, and jot down the bare basics of what you did that day.

It's absurdly easy. Takes about thirty seconds. And if you forget it for a few days, or even a week, you can easily backtrack.

Doing this will have an astonishing effect on your memory of your own life—and, ultimately, on your sense of ownership of it.

When you look back at your calendar, you'll remember a great many things that you would have otherwise forgotten. All it takes is a tiny cue to trigger most memories.

After all, when you were in school, which type of test did you do better on—multiple choice, or fill-in-the-blank? I'm sure you did better on multiple choice. Everyone does. It's easy to be smart when you take a multiple-choice test, because seeing the correct answer usually brings back the memory.

The things you'll write down on your calendar will be the obvious, major things that fill up your life:

- Job activities
- Family activities
- Interactions with friends
- Health
- Travel
- Moods and feelings
- Exercise
- Your weight
- Your fitness achievements
- Problems that arise
- Problems that are solved

When you fill in your calendar, you'll quickly devise your own shorthand system, with lots of abbreviating, because there's not much room in a calendar space. Besides, you don't need all the little details to keep a memory alive. If you just write, "Burned birthday cake," it will bring back more than enough memories.

Abbreviating things, or coding them, also helps keep your private matters private. It helps keep memories in your head, where they belong, instead of out there for all the world to see.

You will soon discover that when you put things in black and white, you can get to the truth of your life a lot more often. For example, you might see that you haven't been exercising enough, even though you might feel like you have been, or you might see that you've only had two fights with your teenage son during the past year, even though he thinks you've been fighting all the time.

You will also discover that when you begin to fill out your calendar, patterns will emerge. As certain events occur again and again, it will, for example, become much more obvious what makes you sick, what makes you worry, what makes you happy, what makes you lose weight, or what makes you skip your exercise. You'll become an expert on you.

You won't always like what you see. But you'll always learn from it.

I have a friend who has been doing this for twenty years. He says that if his house ever caught on fire, his calendars would be the first thing he'd grab, even before his photo albums. For him, his calendars contain a more intimate and accurate "picture" of his life than any group of photos ever could.

To be a whole person, you need to run your own life.

And you'll never really be able to run it unless you know exactly what's happened.

Phase Three | Fitness Element #2 | *Power Food*

Phase Three: Creating a New Life with Power Food

Now you conclude your six-week nutrition makeover with a bang. There are some nutrition elements in Phase Three that are going to make your life better by the end of the day. How's that for a bang?

You deserve this. You did the heavy lifting in Phases One and Two, by changing your basic diet to a common-sense, low-cal, balanced eating plan. That took discipline. Now it's time to add some elements that are easy.

I introduce supplements and formulas in this phase. The purpose of these supplements is to give you a more efficient metabolism, more vitality, a more youthful appearance, and an enhanced ability to transform the food you eat into energy, instead of body fat.

I waited until this phase to add these supplements because I wanted you to know that your progress thus far was not based on any pill, but on your own hard work. Now that you know this, you'll be less tempted to rely too much upon supplements and to blow off good eating habits. People who do that never succeed.

In Phase Three, I'll also help you to fine-tune your diet by introducing the topic of food reactions, including food allergies and the milder food sensitivities. Most people have at least a couple of food sensitivities, but don't even know it. All they know is that they often carry around a puffy, false fat of water weight and bloating, and that they tend to have food cravings. If you have any food sensitivities, you'll soon know what they are. And when you start eliminating the offending foods from your diet, your energy, mood, and fitness levels will rocket.

A word of warning: Don't think that because you've already done the painful part of changing your diet that you've done everything—because things don't have to hurt to help. Many healing factors feel good.

The Fitness Supplement A-List

You cannot achieve peak fitness without taking supplements. It can't be done.

All of my star clients take supplements. No exceptions. Obviously, many of them eat diets that are almost preternaturally perfect. But even these clients need supplements.

The main reason they all take supplements is that a diet that's low in calories rarely has a sufficient volume of foodstuffs to provide a rich, powerful, wide array of micronutrients: vitamins, minerals, enzymes, amino acids, and essential fatty acids. For example, to achieve the amount of vitamin C in just a single one-grain tablet, you'd have to eat about twenty oranges, which would contain about 1,200 calories. Therefore, if you wanted to consume about three grams of vitamin C daily in your diet—a high but reasonable amount—you'd have to eat 3,600 calories per day in just oranges.

Of course, it's easy to get enough nutrients in food alone merely to survive, or to avoid deficiency diseases. You need only about one slice of orange every day to avoid scurvy. But my clients don't want to just avoid disease or to just survive—they want to thrive. They want optimal energy, strong immunity, robust fitness, and the chance to achieve longevity in not only their physically demanding careers, but also in their lives. They're ambitious about their bodies. If you are, too, here's a rundown on the supplements I consider most important to holistic fitness.

Some of them are supplements I helped design myself. For years, I struggled to find brands that were adequate for people who wanted only the best, but it was difficult. Even most of the high-end brands, many of which are overpriced, were lacking in ingredients I felt were vital. For example, I could never find a protein powder that contained extra glutamine, or one that contained essential fatty acids, even though both of these ingredients are necessary for optimal muscle toning. Therefore, I arranged with various supplement suppliers to produce products for me that met my own specifications. I sourced out the world's best suppliers, the people who were really on the cutting edge, and helped them develop the world's finest supplements, customized in very exact formulas. Many of the products my clients now use are from this line. My clients expect nothing but the very best, especially regarding things that they put into their bodies.

The Six Essentials

Protein Complete: organic whey protein with glutamine. It's the most complete organic protein powder available. Three reasons. Number one: It contains an extra 1,200 mg of glutamine, which the muscles need to grow during the crucial post-workout recovery period. Number two: It contains essential fatty acids, which synergistically boost muscle growth. Most manufacturers of protein powder leave out the EFAs because they add calories. Foolish omission. EFAs burn far more calories than they add. Also, studies indicate that EFAs help prevent injuries from exercise, by supporting muscle rebuilding. Number three: The organic whey protein comes from grass-fed cows that feed on chemical-free, pesticide-free, and hormone-free grassland, a breakthrough in quality protein. You'll never go back to conventional powders again. Another thing our protein has that many others don't is the digestive probiotics that increase the body's uptake of protein. This protein powder makes a great snack, because it's pure nutrition, contains fiber, is low-carb, is very filling, and is tasty. No one on a vigorous exercise regimen should neglect taking extra protein. Protein is the only substance that rebuilds and repairs tissues.

Fat Burning Lemonade™ is a product I'm especially proud to have helped develop, because it has the unique action of being a sweet-tasting drink that actually promotes weight loss. It supports the body in the conversion of body fat to energy by gently enhancing metabolic efficiency. It also contains pharmaceutical-grade L-carnitine tartrate, an amino acid that helps shuttle fat out of the system. This is ideal for sugar-free diets because the xylitol and stevia ingredient has a negligible effect on insulin.

Healthy Omega-3 is a pharmaceutical-grade marine lipid concentrate, unlike most omega-3 oils, and is distilled for purity. It not only boosts fat burning, but also younger-looking skin (by, in effect, moisturizing the skin from the inside out). In addition, it magnifies the muscle-toning and fat-burning effects of the Protein Complete powder.

Super Calcium Complex with Hydroxyapatite. Everybody knows bones need calcium, but many people don't realize calcium is vital for proper muscle contraction, a major variable in muscle strength. Your muscles will never feel right, particularly after a workout, if you have even a slight calcium deficit. The hydroxyapatite in this formula, which is absent in most commercial calcium, is the absolute best ingredient for maximizing absorption.

Immune Elixir is a blend of potent herbs that helps the body kill and flush away pathogens, including bacteria, viruses, and fungi. My clients use it to help prevent minor illnesses, and to speed recovery from colds, flu, sinusitis, and symptoms of airborne allergies.

Super Multi-Energy Food is the best "multi" vitamin available, because it's not only a multivitamin/multimineral, but also a multisuperfood and multiherbal. It contains innumerable micronutrients that are generally missing from even healthy diets. Another unique aspect of the formula is the presence of probiotics, which makes the remainder of the formula eminently digestible and absorbable. Unlike almost all other products in the "multi" category, only one tablet per day is needed. Now that's power.

Also on the Honor Roll

- **Alpha lipoic acid** enhances antioxidant functions of vitamin C, vitamin E, and glutathione. It is involved in the conversion of carbohydrates to energy and converts sugar to energy. Useful for energy metabolism. Assists with heavy metal and metabolic detoxification. Also great for diabetes, immune disorders, and liver, heart, and eye disorders.
- **Alpha ketogluteric acid** is essential for carbohydrate metabolism. Dependent on B-vitamins and alpha lipoic acid for activation. This prevents buildup of lactic acid.
- **Cinnamon**—yep, plain old cinnamon—which exerts a notable stabilizing force against blood-sugar fluctuation.
- **Ginseng,** an effective remedy in times of great mental and physical stress, helps the body cope with fatigue. Increases immune function and resistance to infection.
- **Glucosamine and chondroitin** support the health of cartilage, and thereby help prevent sports injuries and arthritic degeneration.
- **Green tea polyphenols** are tremendously rich in antioxidants.
- **Super green super food** supports the five foundations of health, nutrition, digestion, circulation, and immunity. Helps keep the body alkaline.

YOUR TO-DO LIST

1. Comparison shop for supplements. Prices and quality vary drastically. Trust your pharmacist, naturopath, or health-food store proprietor. Err on the side of quality (over cost). If you gain even one extra workday due to disease prevention, your supplements will have paid for themselves.
2. To find the Six Essentials, visit our Web site at www.onebodyonelife.com. The Six Essentials are also available in select stores.

Get a Flat Stomach *Fast!*

You liked the "fast" part, right?

As a rule, I'm contemptuous of fast weight-loss methods, because they invariably trigger rebound weight gain. But there's one way to lose weight quickly without causing a rebound: losing what some doctors now call *false fat*. False fat is the five to ten extra pounds of water weight, generally accompanied by abdominal bloating from gas, that comes from eating foods that cause food reactions. False fat isn't really fat, or adipose tissue, but it looks like fat, feels like fat, and can last forever if you don't do something about it.

Most people think of food reactions as allergies, but allergies are just one type of food reaction. The other, more common type of reaction is a food sensitivity, which is an allergy, but milder. All forms of food reactions, however, have similar symptoms: water retention, abdominal bloating from gas, food cravings, heartburn and indigestion, facial puffiness, and low energy. If you frequently have more than one of these symptoms, it's quite possibly due to food reactions.

Food reactions typically occur when people can't fully digest what they eat. For example, the food reaction of lactose intolerance is an inability to fully digest lactose, the sugar in dairy products. When food molecules can't be fully digested, the body identifies them as foreign invaders—such as pathogens—and tries to get rid of them, in part by washing them away with extra water.

This inability to fully digest foods is extremely common these days, because:

- **We eat too narrow a range of foods.** Most people get about 75 percent of their total calories from only about ten of their favorite staples. Unfortunately, when you overeat any one food, you can exhaust your body's ability to digest it, by depleting specific digestive enzymes.
- **We eat artificial foods** that the body doesn't recognize as foods.
- **We eat foods we're not genetically programmed to eat.** The easiest foods to digest are those your ancestors thrived on. The hardest to digest are the foods your ancestors rarely ate. For example, Asians and African-Americans have extremely high rates of lactose intolerance, mostly because their ancestors didn't consume many dairy products.

Because it's hard for your body to digest foods that you eat too often—"repeat offenders"—the foods that most often cause food reactions are usually very common foods.

THE SIX REPEAT OFFENDERS
1. Wheat
2. Dairy products
3. Eggs
4. Corn
5. Soy
6. Peanuts

Others that often cause problems are shellfish, chocolate, gluten (in wheat, rye, and oats), citrus fruits, MSG, and aspartame.

People often love the foods to which they are most reactive, because reactive foods can cause a druglike response. As they enter the bloodstream—and trigger a distress alarm when they're identified as a foreign invader—part of the body's distress response is a release of feel-good endorphins, and energy-boosting insulin and adrenaline. This creates temporary spikes of contentment and satisfaction—which inevitably subside, causing a desire for more of the food: cravings!

It's easy to find out if you're reactive to various foods by taking a rather expensive doctor's test. Most people, though, can figure it out just by avoiding certain suspicious foods for about a week, to see if their symptoms subside. To do this, restrict all of your suspicious foods—the ones you eat most often, and seem to crave. Then add them back in one at a time, looking for symptoms, such as indigestion, or the gain of water weight. This procedure can be challenging, because it's hard to avoid your favorite foods. But it can really pay off.

When you eliminate all your reactive foods, you'll probably lose several pounds of water weight, or edema, almost instantly. You'll look and feel much better. And after you rid your system of the last vestiges of your offending foods, your cravings for them will drop dramatically. Conquering cravings will benefit your dieting efforts tremendously.

You'll quickly find that there are numerous substitutes available for virtually all foods. Why? Because millions of people need them, since food reactions are so common.

Do You Have Food Reactions?

1. Certain common foods tend to give me indigestion.	**Yes**	**No**
2. Sometimes I get puffy in the face—or my hands swell up a little—for no apparent reason.	**Yes**	**No**
3. I'm just crazy about certain foods. I can't get enough of them.	**Yes**	**No**
4. I occasionally binge eat, but usually on particular foods.	**Yes**	**No**
5. When I get hungry, I usually focus my hunger on a particular favorite food.	**Yes**	**No**
6. I eat more or less the same foods most of the time—not much variety. I like it that way.	**Yes**	**No**
7. I frequently eat foods that I know don't agree with me.	**Yes**	**No**
8. Sometimes special foods—such as chocolate, or even a glass of cold milk—cheer me up.	**Yes**	**No**
9. Certain foods seem to make me go into almost a trance, and when that happens I tend to eat too much of them.	**Yes**	**No**

10.	Sometimes my belly gets bloated even when I don't eat very much.	**Yes**	**No**
11.	Some foods make my nose feel stuffy and congested, as if I have hay fever.	**Yes**	**No**
12.	When I'm hungry, even a small amount of one of my very favorite foods picks me up.	**Yes**	**No**

Score

If you answered yes to even a small number of these questions, such as two or three, it could indicate that you are reactive to specific foods. Don't be too surprised.

Food reactions are much more common than most people realize.

Ten Simple Rules for Dining Out

Rules 1, 2, 3, 4, and 5: Eat like you do at home. Don't eat excess calories just because you're in a restaurant. If you do, you'll end up shunning restaurants. Or you'll end up overweight. There are invariably a number of healthy dishes that are served in virtually every restaurant. Find them. Enjoy them. You'll feel so much better about eating out. You'll end up doing it more often.

Rule 6. Order simple foods. The more elaborate your dish is, the more likely it will be to contain hidden calories. If you can't tell exactly what's on your plate, it will probably be fattening. After all, why shouldn't the chef hide cream, butter, and sugar in his food? His only job is to make the food taste good. He's not your dietician or your trainer.

Rule 7. Skip the bread. At home, you don't sit around for half an hour before dinner eating bread and butter, do you? It's too fattening! If the service is slow and you can't wait to eat, order a salad.

Rule 8. Share your appetizer. Or skip it entirely. Appetizers are almost always higher in calories, per volume, than entrees.

Rule 9. Share your dessert. Or skip it. You wouldn't eat a 600-calorie concoction at home, would you? Great desserts are fun, but like all intense pleasures, they're best in small amounts.

Rule 10. Focus on the things that don't make you fat. The ambiance. Your company. The pleasure of having someone else do all the work.

Remember, dining out can be a very pleasurable, sensually satisfying, and healthy part of your life—or a disaster that you end up avoiding as much as possible.

It's your choice.

SAMPLE RECIPES

• BREAKFAST EXAMPLES •

Recipe 1—Baked Apple and Cinnamon

1 apple

cinnamon to taste

Core apple and sprinkle with cinnamon. Place in small oven and cook slowly. You may top with yogurt.

Recipe 2—Fruit Salad Topped with Yogurt and Seeds

$1/4$ cup strawberries

$1/4$ cup blackberries

1 cup yogurt

1 tbsp each of sunflower seeds, pumpkin seeds

Slice strawberries thinly. Add blackberries. Top with yogurt and seeds. Seeds may be lightly toasted on low heat.

Recipe 3—Toasted Mozzarella and Egg Cracker

1 egg boiled

$1/4$ cup mozzarella cheese

$1/4$ cup each of tomato, mushrooms

2–4 non-yeast, wheat-free crackers

Fry tomato and mushrooms with olive oil cooking spray. Top crackers with boiled egg, tomato, and mushroom. Melt mozzarella cheese on top.

Recipe 4—Egg and Vegetable Scramble

1 egg

$1/3$ cup egg whites

1 tbsp slivered almonds

$1/4$ cup cherry tomatoes

garlic and herbs to taste

2 non-yeast, wheat-free crackers

Sauté slivered almonds on low heat until warm; add cherry tomatoes. Fry egg, egg whites, garlic, and herbs in separate pan. Mix all ingredients together as a scramble.

Recipe 5—Turkey or Tofu Scramble

$^1/_2$ cup egg whites
4 ounces sliced turkey breast or tofu
garlic and herbs to taste

Sauté egg whites with sliced turkey or tofu. Add herbs. May be placed on top of non-yeast, wheat-free cracker.

• LUNCH EXAMPLES •

Recipe 1—Beef Burger with Vegetables, or Stir-fry Beef

4–6 ounces extra lean ground beef
$^1/_4$ cup each of tomato, mushroom, green pepper
garlic and herbs to taste

Mold ground beef into burger patty. Fry burger patty in frying pan using olive oil spray until brown. Add tomato, mushroom, and green pepper to same pan until soft. Or: Brown ground beef in frying pan using the olive oil spray; add garlic and herbs. Then add finely chopped vegetables to pan, lower heat, and simmer for 5 to 10 minutes.

Recipe 2—Tuna Salad

1 can tuna (canned in water/drained)
1 tbsp olive oil (extra-virgin, cold-pressed)
1 lemon to taste
4 olives
onion, garlic, sea salt to taste
basil, parsley to taste
salad greens, as much as you like

Toss together all ingredients. Serve over green salad.

Recipe 3—Lemon Almond Chicken with Green Beans

> 4–6 ounces chicken breast
>
> 1 lemon to taste
>
> paprika, sea salt to taste
>
> 1 cup green beans
>
> 1 tbsp slivered almonds

Season chicken breast with flavoring and lemon. Place in oven. Bake at 200 degrees for 15 minutes. Steam green beans. Toast slivered almonds until golden brown. Top chicken and green beans with toasted slivered almonds.

Recipe 4—Vegetable Bake

> 1 cup each of cauliflower, broccoli, or as much as you like
>
> 1/4 cup mozzarella cheese
>
> sea salt to taste

Boil or steam vegetables. Top with mozzarella cheese and place in oven to allow cheese to melt and brown.

• DINNER EXAMPLES •

Recipe 1—Lemon-Crusted Snapper

> 4–6 ounces snapper
>
> 1 lemon to taste
>
> 2–4 non-yeast, wheat-free crackers
>
> herbs, sea salt to taste
>
> salad greens, as much as you like

Squeeze lemon over snapper. Add herbs and sea salt. Crumb the crackers and sprinkle onto fish. Place snapper in ovenproof dish with olive oil spray. Cook in oven at 180 degrees for 15 minutes. Serve over salad greens.

Recipe 2—Beef Stew

> 4–6 ounces beef, lean
>
> 1 cup spinach, or as much as you like
>
> 1/2 cup each of tomato, onion
>
> garlic, paprika, sea salt to taste

Brown onions and beef using olive oil spray. Add ½ cup boiling water or vegetable broth (see condiments). Add garlic, paprika, and sea salt, and bring to boil. Reduce heat and simmer 20 minutes, stirring occasionally. Add spinach and tomato, and simmer until the liquid is reduced by one-third.

Recipe 3—Capsicum Bake

4–6 ounces extra lean ground beef
$^1/_4$ cup onions
garlic, parsley, sea salt to taste
$^1/_2$ cup each of capsicum, mushrooms
$^1/_4$ cup mozzarella cheese

Brown onions and ground beef in a pan, using an olive oil spray. Add mushrooms, garlic, parsley, and sea salt. Fill capsicum with cooked mixture. Top with cheese and place in oven. Bake until cooked.

Recipe 4—Chicken Curry Kebab Sticks

4–6 ounces chicken breast, skinned
$^1/_2$ cup each of mushroom, cherry tomato, zucchini
1 each of apple, mango
curry powder, garlic, sea salt to taste
1 tbsp olive oil (extra-virgin, cold-pressed)

Cube chicken, zucchini, apple, and mango into a large bowl. Add mushrooms and cherry tomatoes. Coat all the ingredients with olive oil, curry powder, garlic, and sea salt. Marinate for 10 minutes in refrigerator. Skewer a piece of chicken with a mushroom, cherry tomato, zucchini, and piece of apple and mango on a kebab stick. Cook on barbeque for 5 to 10 minutes, until chicken is cooked.

Recipe 5—Turkey Salad

4–6 ounces turkey breast, skinned
lettuce, watercress, as much as you like
$^1/_2$ cup each of tomato, cucumber, snow peas, or as much as you like
2 tbsp avocado
1 tbsp olive oil (extra-virgin, cold-pressed)

Slice turkey breast. Shred lettuce. Chop tomatoes, cucumber, and avocado. Add watercress and snow peas. Toss everything in a bowl. Top with olive oil. You may substitute turkey with another low-fat protein source.

Recipe 1—Cracker and Cottage Cheese

$1/4$ cup cottage cheese (low-fat)
tomato, cucumber, scallions, lettuce, as much as you like
2–4 non-yeast, wheat-free crackers

Slice tomato and cucumber. Place tomato, cucumber, scallions, lettuce, and cottage cheese on crackers.

Recipe 2—Cheese Dip and Vegetable Crudités

$1/4$ cup cream cheese, light
$1/2$ cup each of carrot, celery, broccoli, cauliflower
herbs and spices to taste

Mix cream cheese with herbs and spices to taste to make a dip. Boil vegetables 1 to 3 minutes, drain, and plunge into ice water. Drain; pat dry. You may add non-yeast, wheat-free crackers.

Recipe 3—Bean Dip and Vegetable Crudités

$1/2$ cup red kidney beans
$1/4$ cup cream cheese, light
1 lemon to taste
$1/2$ cup each of carrot, celery, broccoli, cauliflower
herbs and spices to taste

Mix red kidney beans, cream cheese, and lemon with a little water. Add herbs and spices to taste to make a dip. Boil vegetables 1 to 3 minutes, drain, and plunge into ice water. Drain; pat dry. You may add non-yeast, wheat-free crackers.

Recipe 4—Vegetarian Pizza

2–4 non-yeast, wheat-free crackers
onions, capsicum, zucchini, tomatoes, mushrooms, as much as
   you like
garlic, mixed herbs to taste
$1/4$ cup ricotta cheese, or mozzarella cheese

Stir-fry all vegetables with garlic and mixed herbs with an olive oil spray. Place vegetables on non-yeast, wheat-free crackers and top with cheese. Bake in oven for 1 minute, and serve.

Recipe 5—Trail Mix

$^1/_2$ cup sunflower seeds
$^1/_2$ cup pumpkin seeds
$^1/_2$ cup sesame seeds
10 almonds

Sauté all ingredients on low heat for 2 minutes until golden brown while stirring. You may flavor it with tamari, or add sea salt. This recipe makes 2 servings.

• CONDIMENT EXAMPLES •

Recipe 1—Almond Butter Sauce

2 tbsp almond butter
1 lemon to taste
3 tbsp tamari
chili, garlic, ginger, sea salt to taste

Heat almond butter and water in a small saucepan over medium heat. Add lemon, tamari, chili, garlic, ginger, and sea salt to taste. Simmer uncovered, for sauce to thicken.

Recipe 2—Tahini Dressing

$^1/_4$ cup tahini
$^1/_4$ cup yogurt (optional)
1 lemon to taste
1–3 tbsp tamari
1 tbsp chili (optional)

Mix equal parts of tahini with equal parts of yogurt, or water, into a dressing. Add lemon, chili, and tamari to taste.

Recipe 3—Tamari Dipping Sauce

3 tbsp tamari (Watch tamari daily allowance.)
$^1/_4$ cup scallions (green onion)
1 tbsp sesame oil
garlic, ginger, chili to taste

Mix tamari and sliced scallions in a bowl. Add sesame oil, garlic, ginger, and chili to taste.

Recipe 4—Vegetable Broth

1/2 cup each of celery, onion, mushroom

1/4 cup each of parsley, bay leaves

garlic to taste

Boil vegetables until tender. Add flavoring. Simmer for 30 minutes. Strain and discard vegetables and retain broth. Freeze for later use.

• SHAKE EXAMPLES •

Recipe 1—Berry Yogurt Shake

1/2 cup blueberries, fresh or frozen

1/2 cup raspberries, fresh or frozen

1 cup yogurt, nonfat

1 tsp flaxseed oil

1–2 scoops Protein Complete powder

Blend all ingredients in blender. Option: add ice.

Recipe 2—Morning Energizer Shake

1 date

1/2 cup blueberries, fresh or frozen

1 cup unsweetened vanilla soy milk

1/2 tbsp raw almond butter

1–2 scoops Protein Complete powder

Blend all ingredients in blender. Option: add ice.

Recipe 3—Mango Peach Shake

1/2 cup mango, fresh or frozen

1/2 cup peach, fresh or frozen

1 tbsp almond butter

1–2 scoops Protein Complete powder

1 oz cranberry juice, unsweetened

8 oz water

Blend all ingredients in blender. Option: add ice.

Phase Three | **Fitness Element #3** | *Cleansing*

Phase Three: Creating a New Life with Cleansing

How's this for short?

Do the Weekend Cleanse again—on both Saturday and Sunday.

That's your entire Phase-Three cleansing.

Can't get much shorter than that, can you?

You've come a long way, and you've learned a lot. You don't need much more information. You are so close to the end of this program that what you mostly need now is action.

The two-day Weekend Cleanse will give you plenty of action. It will be a bit more challenging than the one-day Weekend Cleanse that you did in Phase Two, but that challenge will pay dividends in forty-eight hours. By the end of this two-day Weekend Cleanse, you'll feel cleaner, fresher, and lighter than you have in a long time.

For all the details on the Weekend Cleanse, review the material in Phase Two. You do exactly the same thing—but this time you do it for two days in a row.

Because you'll be eating less than usual, you may wish to cut back somewhat on your physical activity. This may not be the best time for a nice weekend hike, or for swimming at the beach. Just relax, get some sun and fresh air if you can, and enjoy the fact that you've come so far!

Phase Three | **Fitness Element #4** | *Exercise*

Phase Three: Creating a New Life with Exercise

I hope you're ready for some high-action, really enjoyable work. After a month in the trenches of fitness, you should be. You're probably not the same person you were a month ago. You're undoubtedly stronger, tougher—and more ready to tackle a challenge than you've ever been.

In all probability, your body has already begun to change, but now you're going to start seeing new changes almost every day. The increased intensity and the extra reps in these Phase-Three Workouts will accelerate your sculpting, toning, and fat loss, as your new body becomes your permanent body.

Get addicted to the work. Make a choice to love it. Get into it!

You have only one more level to go. Soon you'll be at the summit, doing hard work as if it were easy. This happens all the time. It will happen to you.

To Get Maximum Benefits from Each Rep:
Feel the Muscle, Not the Weight

Sometimes when I look at people who are exercising, I can see an image of what's going on inside of them. I can often see this image so clearly that it's almost as if they're casting a shadow of their inner self on the wall.

For example, I'll see a guy who is in decent shape, lifting a weight with relatively good form, and as I look at him, his shadow emerges. It's the shadow of a man going through his finances, struggling and straining. His shadow is saying, "My financial burden is more important than my body."

It's very clear that he's fragmented, disconnected, not into his body and not into his breath. He's just going through the motions, while his mind is preoccupied with things he thinks are more important than his own body.

And I just want to shake a guy like this by the shoulders, and say, "Get connected—get out of your head and into your body."

I want him to feel his body, not the weight of his problems. If you feel your body, you're building a relationship with your true self. If you feel the weight, you're building a relationship with drudgery.

Lots of people just don't get it when they work out. They're focused on the distant future, on that make-believe time when they'll look perfect, and life will be easy. Forget that!

Everything you need is right here.

When you gain the power to change your experience, you can change everything. Changing your body will just be the beginning!

Start by feeling the muscle, not the weight.

The Joy of Exercising Outside

Most people seem to primarily work out indoors these days. That's okay for most people. For me, I'd rather be outside.

As far as I'm concerned, my body and the world that surrounds it are one and the same. When I get connected with my body during a workout, I also want to get connected to the earth. I suppose this feeling is a residual effect of the Aloha Spirit that I grew up with.

In my opinion, there's nothing like the physical rush you get from running barefoot in the sand, with the wind cooling you and the sun warming you. And I don't think that any stair-stepper in the world can provide the exhilaration you get from climbing a steep, green hill, dotted with rocks and wildflowers. There's no piece of gym equipment ever made that can evoke the primal satisfaction you get from doing landscape work in your own yard.

When you're exercising outdoors, you drink in nature's chi like an elixir of pure energy.
You forget that you're working out, because you're not working: You're playing.
You connect to the kid you once were.
You connect to the earth.
You connect to your self.

Back to Breath

The more in touch you are with your breath, the more you will achieve from your workout.

<blockquote>

If your goals and your intention are clear—

and if they connect to your body through your breath—

you will see results manifest quickly.

Too Many People Tune Out.
YOU MUST DIAL IN!

To do it: Just connect to the body . . . AND BREATHE!
Everything starts with the breath.

</blockquote>

What's the Maximum Time to Exercise?

Don't ask me. Ask your body.

If you're really connected to your body, it will tell you exactly when to stop.

There is no universal rule on the maximum amount of time you should work out. There isn't even a limit on the maximum number of reps you should do of any particular exercise.

In fact, here's a little secret. Don't tell my clients—but I hate counting reps. I think the numbers of reps that people do are mostly meaningless. I can't tell you how many times I've gotten busted by my clients for not counting their reps correctly. I'll be going, "And twenty, and twenty-one, and twenty-two, and twenty-three, and twenty-three, and twenty-four," and the client will shoot me a look, like, "Yo, Greg! You awake?"

Sure I'm awake. But I'm focusing on their breath, and their form, and how they're connecting, and how their muscles are responding—not on the number of reps.

Connect to how you feel. Feel the muscle, not the weight. When you do that, you can bust right past your required twenty-five reps, and hit thirty-five. Or fifty. Whatever.

Just keep going. Go for the flow, and let its current run through you. Don't do two minutes and then disconnect. Don't do five minutes and disconnect. Do the full half-hour, and then wake up from it as if from a dream.

When that happens, you'll go, "Wow! I hit my stride today! I changed my body! I own it! I get it! It's Buddha Time!"

And my reaction to that invariably is: "Well, hello there! I've been waiting for you! Welcome to holistic fitness!"

If you can reach this level of being plugged in to your body, you'll probably never run a serious risk of overtraining or overstraining. You'll know when to say when.

But we all get carried away sometimes, don't we? Occasionally we just overdo it. So here are the six major signs that you've pushed yourself too hard, and that you need to scale down your basic workout program:

THE SIX WARNING SIGNS OF EXCESSIVE EXERCISE

1. **You suffer from extended loss of appetite.**
2. **Even when you're at rest, your heart rate is slightly elevated above its usual level.**
3. **You experience a mild mood disturbance, such as anxiety or depression, for no apparent reason.**
4. **You have persistent muscle pain, even when you don't exercise very hard.**
5. **Even after a day of rest, you still feel fatigued.**
6. **You have nagging injuries that just won't heal.**

If you notice any of these signs, give yourself a break. Either back off considerably from your exercise program, or stop completely and rest for at least a few days. Then start in again gradually.

It's true: You've only got one body. But you've only got one life, too—and the point of life is to live it, not just endure it.

So when your body says "stop"—stop.

Chapter 7

Into the Future

Now, for week seven.

Yes, there is a week seven. And a week eight, nine, ten, eleven, twelve—you get the idea. A program as valuable as this should never end.

You can't let this program end. As Bob Dylan once wrote, "If you ain't busy being born, you're busy dying." The same principle applies to fitness: If you aren't busy getting fit, you're busy getting fat. There is no middle ground. Use it or lose it.

During weeks seven, eight, nine—and beyond—you must continue to exercise on the same five-days-per-week basis. You do not need to keep doing the challenging Phase-Three Workouts, particularly when your energy is low. You can alternate them with the easier workouts. If you try to do too much, you run the risk of burnout.

You may also, at this point, begin to mix and match your favorite forms of these workouts. If you love Pilates Day and hate Yoga Day, go ahead and do more Pilates. Remember, though, that you must have some variation in your workouts in order to hit all your muscle groups.

In addition, now that you have a solid base of fitness, you may start to integrate many other physical activities into your program of exercise: hiking, weight lifting, skiing, dancing, swimming, jogging, tennis, bicycling, basketball, golf, skating, rowing—anything that gets you moving, and breathing, and stretching, and working.

Don't skimp: Do the full thirty minutes. Varying your exercise is no excuse to start cutting yourself slack. If you do less than thirty minutes per day, five times each week, your fitness will begin to erode. Honor the power of the Magic Half-Hour.

Also, you must continue to eat a wholesome, healthy diet, moderate in fat and carbs. This means, eat a diet based around lean meat, high-fiber vegetables, a moderate amount of whole grains, fruits, and essential fats. This combination of food will give you power.

You need never be hungry. Power food, even in relative abundance, almost always helps your body more than it hurts it. Just don't go overboard and start cramming calories just for fun. Continue to feed your body, not your mouth.

You've also got to keep your mind and spirit working for you, instead of against you. Review the mind and spirit sections often. The advice in them is like all other good advice: easy to give, but hard to accept. Your ongoing task is to accept this advice, and work it into your life. Don't just learn it—live it.

And, of course, you've got to do your best to stay away from toxins, and to get rid of them when they invade. Do the cleansing program on a regular basis—every few weeks would be excellent. Stay intimately aware of the health and function of your organs of elimination, particularly your liver, kidneys, skin, colon, and lymphatic system. If any of these areas seem to need help, nurture them. This will help keep you young.

So, as you see, this new way of living will never end. But at this point—after the changes you've made in your body and your life—you shouldn't want it to end, because the process of fitness is even more gratifying than the product. It's the day-to-day process of fitness—the working out, the power-eating, the cleansing, and the focusing—that feels so good.

This never-ending need for action is the burden of fitness. And the blessing.

Embrace this burden. Celebrate this blessing.

If you do, you will be able to look at yourself in the mirror each morning and say, "I have changed."

You will know without need of any other evidence that you have grown.

Maybe you started out on this program thinking, "Gee, I wouldn't mind looking like a movie star in six weeks!" But that was the old you. The one who had not yet done the work that movie stars do.

Now you've done that work, and it cannot help but have changed you. Now you probably feel at least a little bit more like a movie star—a fantasy figure, above the fray, if only for thirty minutes a day—just as that same work invariably makes movie stars feel more like you, a mere mortal who must always struggle, and fight the urge to quit.

Work is the great equalizer. It humbles the exalted, and exalts the humble.

If you ever happened to meet one of my movie-star clients, you would have a lot to talk about. You'd talk about what it's like to hit the wall that lies beyond will in the Breakthrough

Moment. You'd talk about the pure joy of hurdling that wall with what little strength you have left. You'd talk about things like focus, living in your muscles, staying conscious, the power of breath, cutting slack, being present, doing it right, and building a relationship with yourself. These are the things I talk to the stars about, and these are the things that I've been talking to you about.

If somehow, for some reason, you ever do have occasion to speak to one of these stars, I doubt that, at this point, you would even be intimidated by their fame and fortune. It's true: They really are larger than life. But it's not because they got lucky in Hollywood; it's because they did the work that makes luck happen. You, now, have also done that work. You, like they, are now larger than your own life.

In the final analysis, no matter what our station or status, we all have so much in common: We have all experienced love and loss. We all have but one body, and one life. And we are all mortal.

These are the rock-hard facts of life that bring us all pain, but can also inspire great pride—if we meet these limitations with courage, vigor, and awareness.

You have already done this.

You will continue.

You have gained too much to give up.

Now, at the end, then, I will say to you the same simple thing that I say to my clients after they have, during one more tough workout, enlarged their lives even a bit more.

Well done, my friend!

Well done.

Part

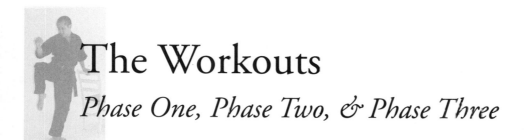

The Workouts

Phase One, Phase Two, & Phase Three

Three

The Phase One Workouts

Welcome to the Phase One Workouts

Do you hate doing the same thing every day?

I do. It gets boring. Your body gets accustomed to the same movements, and stops developing.

You've got to keep changing.

That's why I'm giving you the same kind of varied, multifaceted workout program I give my superstar clients, one that includes a different type of workout each day.

Here's your schedule. It's designed to alternate more demanding days with more restorative days.

1. **Monday: Strength Training**
2. **Tuesday: Yoga**
3. **Wednesday: Pilates**
4. **Thursday: Martial Arts**
5. **Friday: Core Interval Training**

You'll never get bored. And you won't have a single muscle in your body that we won't hit.

Don't worry if you're not familiar with these disciplines.

- **You don't need to be an expert.** Just follow the simple, step-by-step instructions.
- **You do the same basic exercises in all three phases.** Once you learn them in Phase One, your learning curve is over. The last two phases just add a little intensity.

Over the next six weeks:

You'll get stronger.
You'll get more flexible.
You'll get thinner.
You'll get more toned.
You'll get sexier.
You'll get better endurance.

With a bit of work, you'll end up looking like a movie star. That's not out of the realm of possibility. It's up to you.

These workouts are all designed to last for thirty minutes, but because of individual variances, none of them will probably last for exactly thirty minutes. The important thing is to do at least a half-hour. If you finish the exercises before a half-hour has elapsed, repeat some of them. If you're not quite finished with all the exercises in thirty minutes, you may stop.

These workouts were designed in conjunction with some of the brightest minds in the world of physical training—including Irma Joujon-Roche, Steven Ho, Tanja Djelevic, and Yumi Lee: stars in their own right. These masters of physical fitness have helped me train the biggest stars in Hollywood.

You're next.

Now, let's get to the fun part: action!

Phase One | **Monday** | *Strength Training Day*

We begin our week of five workouts with Strength Training Day. Why? Because Strength Day is probably the most strenuous and impactful workout. So let's establish some muscle, start burning fat, and get our results as fast as we can!

Strength Training is the heart and soul of fitness. It not only achieves many of the same benefits as aerobic training—such as improved blood pressure and reduced body fat—but is also the quickest and most direct way to build muscle mass, sculpt the body, and increase bone mineral density.

Here are the most fundamental effects of Strength Training:

- Strength Training halts the loss of muscle mass during aging. Without exercise people average a loss of about five to seven pounds of muscle every decade. This can not only be arrested, but reversed.
- Strength Training has a profound cardiovascular impact. It is virtually as effective as aerobic exercise at regulating blood pressure. During Strength Training sessions, systolic blood pressure increases by 35 to 50 percent, and this results in an enduring reduction of blood pressure.
- The increased muscle mass that comes from Strength Training results in increased metabolic efficiency. Following a session of Strength Training, the "afterburn effect" of increased calorie burning lasts for several hours. In addition, every three pounds of added muscle mass increases the metabolic rate by approximately 7 percent, resulting in an increased daily caloric requirement of about 15 percent.

Despite these wondrous effects, though, only about 5 percent of the American public regularly engages in strenuous Strength Training—about half the number of people who do strenuous aerobic training.

Make yourself part of that elite 5 percent. Those are the people who really look great. Strength Training shows.

Conventional wisdom says that you need fancy machines and big weights to build strength. You can also get fantastic results by using your body's own weight for resistance, along with a few dumbbells. Smart Strength Training is about isolating the power of your focus to hit the exact muscles you need to hit.

You will also find that extra reps—instead of extra weight—are excellent for toning your muscles, with far less risk of injury.

WARM-UP

Go cardio: Get your heart rate up. Nothing fancy. Slow jogging will work. So will fast walking. Hill walking. Treadmill. Stationary bike. Swimming. Ellipticals. Recumbent bike. Just get your heart pumping.

How long: Do 10–15 minutes—just enough to work up a little sweat, loosen your muscles, and open your lungs.

Try to increase your heart rate by about 50 percent. If it's normally about 80 beats per minute when you're at rest, push it up to about 120. This is high enough to kick-start the fat-burning process and get your adrenaline going.

Then shift into these eight exercises. They're challenging. But they'll change your body.

The 30-Minute Workout

These workouts, as I mentioned, are designed to take 30 minutes. But you have your own natural pace. It can even vary from day to day.

Don't rush! It's better to do them right than quickly.

Rest Period Between Sets: It should be dictated by your own energy level. If you're out of breath, take a little extra time to recover. If you feel good: Go!

If part of your body feels tweaked or tight, stretch it out, breathe it out, and take your time before continuing.

Remember: This is your time.

SPECIAL NOTE: As you follow the photos of the exercises, the sequence is from left to right, and then down.

I. SUPERMANS

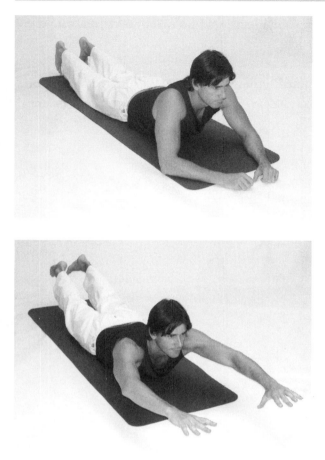

Target: Your butt. Your lower stomach. To a lesser extent, this also targets your entire torso, your upper legs, and your shoulders.

How-To: Lie on a mat or carpet, as pictured, and lift your body as if you were Superman, flying. Focus on the thought of keeping everything but your belly button off the floor. As you lower yourself, squeeze your butt and your triceps. You'll do a lot of squeezing in these exercises, because it doubles the exertion. It combines the isometric exercise of squeezing with the resistance exercise of lifting.

How Long: Do a 30-second hold, 3 times, for a total of 1½ minutes. If that's too hard, break up your 30-second segments into 15-second segments, or even 10-second segments.

The Details:

▶ DO: Be careful. Don't strain your back.
▶ DO: Keep your legs slightly bent, so the effort goes into your muscles, instead of getting locked up in your joints.
▶ DO: Spread your fingers to relax your neck.
▶ DO: Point your feet toes-down, to help keep your body flat.
▶ DON'T: Lock your knees. It reduces muscle involvement.
▶ DON'T: Stop breathing. Take a big breath as you extend, then let it out slowly.
▶ DON'T: Breathe from your throat, but from your belly.

2. SIDE BRIDGES

Target: Your obliques (the muscles on the sides of your abdomen). Your butt. Your back muscles. All of these muscles will coordinate with your abs to help flatten your stomach.

How-To: Lift your body into the position that's pictured, using your elbow and forearm for support. Feet should be heel-to-heel. As you hold it, pull your stomach in tight and squeeze your butt, focusing on that little area where the dimple is.

How Long: Hold it for 30 seconds on each side.

The Details:
▶ DO: Try to keep your body as straight as possible.
▶ DO: Visualize your stomach, sides, and butt, tightening as you squeeze.
▶ DON'T: Let your butt sag.
▶ DON'T: Put tension in your shoulder. This isn't a shoulder exercise. Work your sides.
▶ DON'T: Rely on just one arm if this is too hard. Put your other hand down, as pictured.
▶ DON'T: Hold tension in your neck.

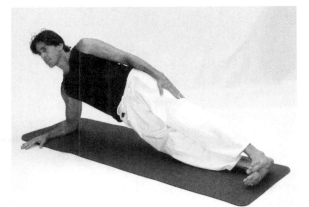

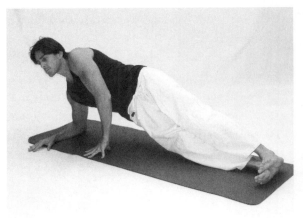

3. PULLOVERS

Target: Your upper abs. (This is a strength move, creating power and stamina, and also a gymnastics move, creating coordination. All of this comes from your abs.)

How-To: Lie on your back, as pictured, and lift your legs and arms at the same time, focusing all the effort on your abs. Go up on a 2-count and down on a 5-count.

How Many: 10 to 20. If you can hit 20, go for it.

The Details:

▶ DO: Squeeze your stomach, tucking it in, as you lift yourself and lower yourself.

▶ DO: Keep your fingers spread, to move tension out of your neck.

▶ DO: Focus. Live in your abs. This move is not about the reps. It's about doing it right.

▶ DON'T: Arch your back. Keep it flat.

▶ DON'T: Crane your neck up. Keep your eyes on the ceiling.

▶ DON'T: Move your knees, hold them in the bent position.

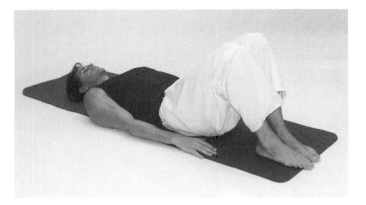

(continued on next page)

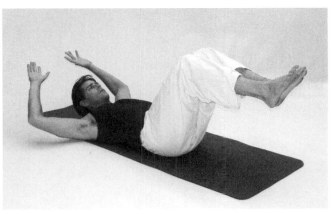

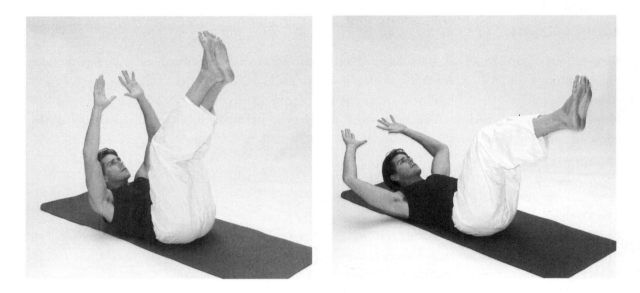

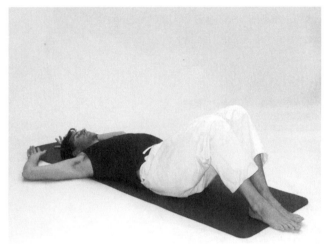

4. TOTAL PUSH-UPS

Target: Everything. The whole body. That's why they're called "total" push-ups.

How-To: Begin in a push-up position then push back (toward your heels). Let your toes grip the ground. Then, as you come back down, swoop forward, as if you were trying to crawl under a fence. That forward-swooping movement is the reason the Navy SEALs call this a Dive Bomber Push-up. Go all the way down, so that your upper body and belly are almost scraping the ground.

How Many: 5 is a good start. 10 is better. If you have to do them in segments, that's okay.

The Details:
- ▶ DO: Stretch your abs and lower back—really open them up.
- ▶ DO: Squeeze your butt as you come up.
- ▶ DO: Point your pinkie outward, and spread your fingers, to take the tension out of your neck, and put it into your triceps and rear deltoids.
- ▶ DON'T: Hyperextend your back—this is all about squeezing and flexing.

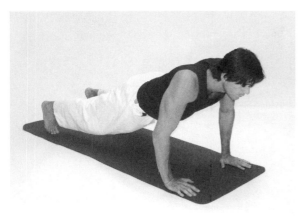

(continued on next page)

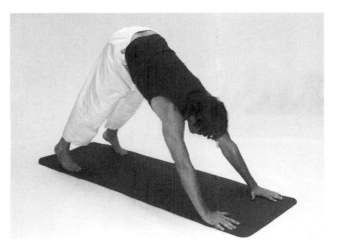

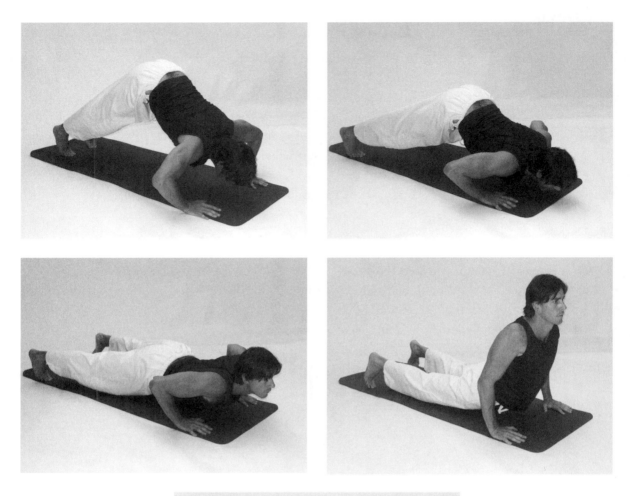

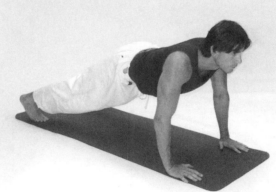

5. OUTSIDE BICEP CURL

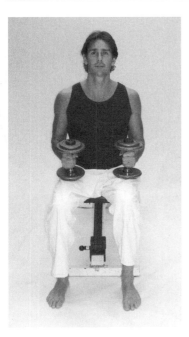

Target: The entire bicep. But this mostly hits the inside line of your arm. It makes it look slender, toned, and sexy.

How-To: Sit on a chair, bed, or weight bench, or sit on the floor on your heels. Sit straight, palms out, with your elbows pressing into your hips. Grip a dumbbell in each hand. (Dumbbells are cheap, easy to find, and the only equipment you'll need for your strength workout.) Men: 10 to 15 pounds. Women: 3¹/₂ to 10 pounds. Use the amount of weight that feels challenging, but comfortable. Lift both weights at once, exhaling on a 2-count lift, and inhaling on a 5-count as the weights go down.

How Many: 3 sets of 20

The Details:

▶ DO: Squeeze your pinkie into the dumbbell, not your thumb, to direct the exertion to your inside bicep, instead of your neck.

▶ DON'T: Keep your elbows on your sides and let them naturally lift away.

▶ DON'T: Put your elbow behind your hip. That puts too much exertion on your shoulder's front delt. Keep the exertion in your bicep.

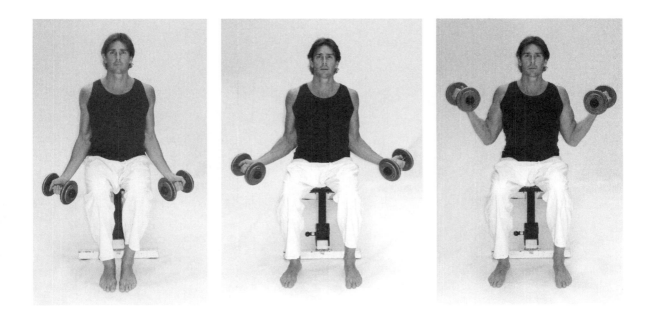

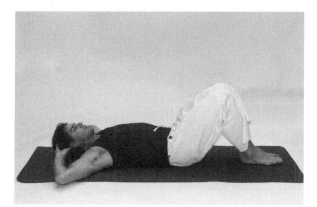

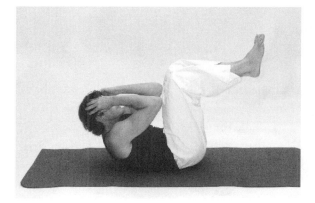

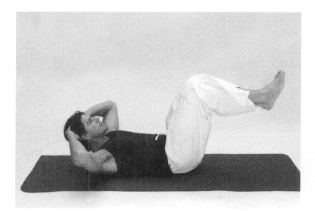

Target: Your abs and the ancillary muscles of your abdomen.

How-To: Lie down as pictured, and put your thumbs by your ears, without interlacing your fingers. Your elbows stay to your sides, your knees are bent, and your feet are flat. Walk your feet out until your toes feel as if they want to come off the ground, and stop right there. Then do a sit-up motion at the same time you bring your knees up, touching your knees with your elbows.

How Many: 3 sets of 15

The Details:

▶ DO: Relax your fingers and neck.
▶ DO: Stay conscious. Don't check out.
▶ DO: Exhale on up, and inhale on down.
▶ DON'T: Arch your back.
▶ DON'T: Bring your chin into your chest. Keep your eyes on the ceiling.
▶ DON'T: Extend your neck, to make it easier to touch your knees. That's cheating. Make your abs do the work.

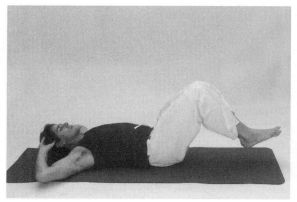

For Women Only: Greg's Lower-Body Blast

This Women-Only Blast is a three-part set of exercises.

7A. PELVIC THRUSTS

Target: Your lower stomach, the outside glutes of your butt, and your hamstrings.

How-To: Come off the ground as pictured. Keep your hands flat, your feet flat, and lift.

How Many: 20. On the 10th and 20th reps, hold it for 10 seconds.

The Details:
- ▶ DO: Go slowly, to keep the work in your butt, and not your back or your knees.
- ▶ DO: Squeeze your butt during the entire exercise.
- ▶ DON'T: Make a fist. It will push the tension to your neck.
- ▶ DON'T: Bounce. That puts the exertion in your joints, not your muscles.
- ▶ DON'T: Arch your lower back—you might strain it.

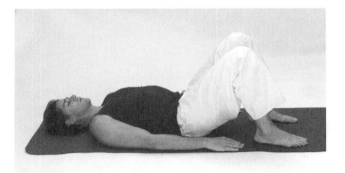

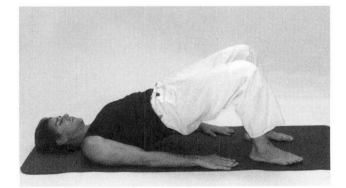

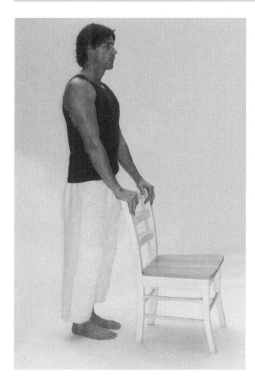

Target: Your outside thighs, upper butt, and calves.

How-To: Use a chair for support, as pictured, with both hands on it, legs together and straight. Lift one leg up and out (or diagonally, halfway between your back and side). Bring it as high as possible—without straining your back. Point your toes down, to create flexion in your butt. Then do the other leg.

How Many: 20 reps with each leg

The Details:

▶ DO: Move with power. Come up quickly, almost as if you were kicking.

▶ DO: Move in super slow-motion as you come down.

▶ DON'T: Let your foot touch the ground. You'll lose your tension.

▶ DON'T: Bounce or hyperextend your leg. If you go too high, your exertion will go to your back, not your butt.

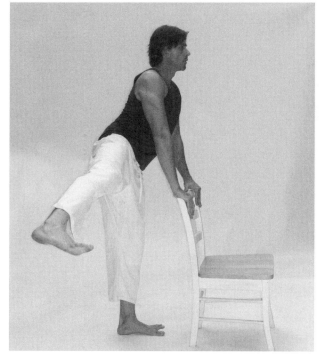

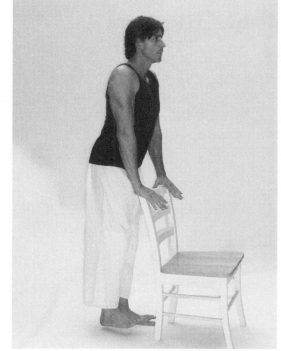

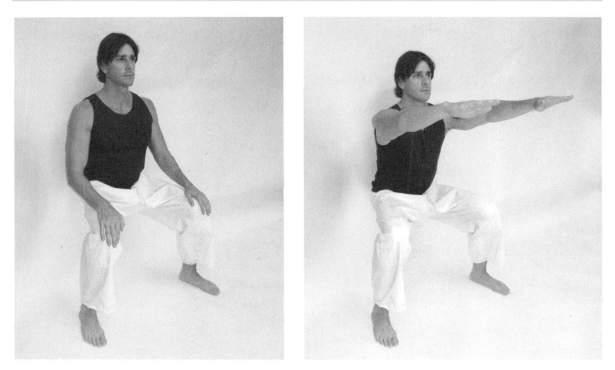

Target: Your inside thighs. Your butt.

How-To: Stand with your back to the wall, as pictured. Lower yourself, using the wall for support, to just below parallel to the ground. Keep your arms out, with your hands a little above parallel. Hold that position.

How Long: Hold it for 45 seconds. Do it in increments if you have to.

The Details:
- ▶ DO: Tuck your stomach in.
- ▶ DO: Keep the exercise in your butt, by keeping your knees behind and in line with your toes.
- ▶ DON'T: Go too low, or the exertion will go to your thighs.
- ▶ DON'T: Make a fist.
- ▶ DON'T: Tense up. If you get tight, wiggle your toes and fingers, or make a sound, to release tension.

For Men Only: Greg's Upper-Body Blast

This Men-Only Blast is a set of three exercises, intended specifically to build upper-body muscle mass.

8A. SUPER TRICEP SKULL-CRUSHERS

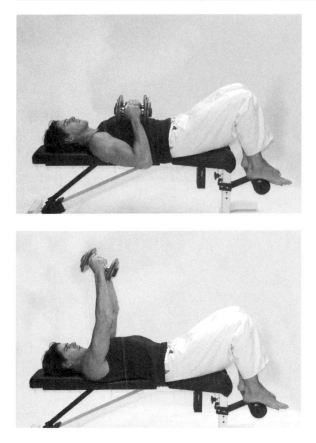

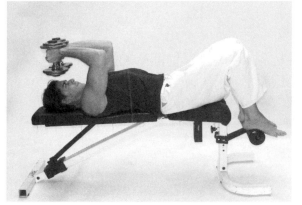

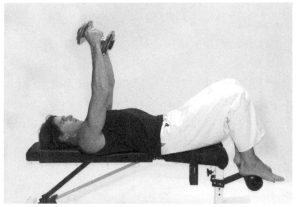

Target: Your triceps.

How-To: Get into the position that's pictured, with 10–15-pound dumbbells, and push your arms straight up. Go down on a count of 5 seconds, and up for 2. Squeeze as you lift.

How Many: 15 reps with 10–15 pounds

The Details:

▶ DO: Keep your palms facing each other, and let them touch if you need a little extra support.

▶ DO: Exhaust your triceps. Focus. Live in your triceps.

▶ DON'T: Squeeze with your thumb. Squeeze with your pinkie.

▶ DON'T: Let your mind wander. Keep it on your triceps.

Target: Your chest.

How-To: With your palms facing each other, make sure your wrist points are outside your elbow points, almost as if you're hugging a barrel. Bring the weights parallel to the ground, and squeeze back up.

How Many: 3 sets of 10 with 10–15 pounds

The Details:
▶ DO: Squeeze the weights on the way up.
▶ DON'T: Let your elbows rest on the ground—just "kiss" it.
▶ DON'T: Squeeze with your thumb—squeeze with your pinkie, to keep your neck out of it.

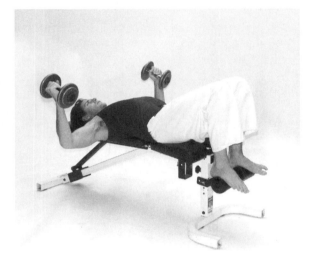

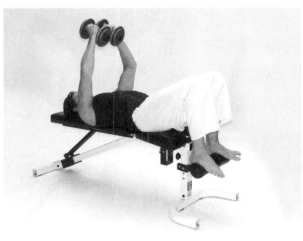

Target: Your chest.

How-To: Lie on your back, as pictured, with 10–15-pound dumbbells out to your sides, shoulder-width apart. Then press up. Squeeze your chest throughout the exercise.

How Many: Do them until your chest or arms start to burn—a minimum of 20.

The Details:
- ▶ DO: Squeeze especially hard as the dumbbells touch.
- ▶ DON'T: Tuck your chin into your chest. It'll make your neck sore.
- ▶ DON'T: Bounce as you come down. That's cheating. Do it right.
- ▶ DON'T: Arch your back. You might tweak it.

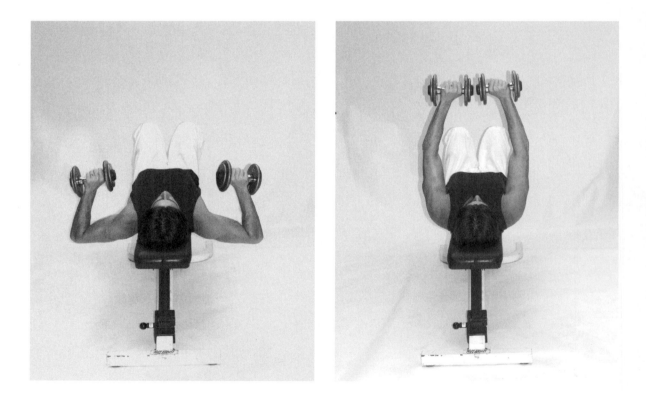

COOLDOWN

After all of your workouts, including the Monday strength workout, you should try to do approximately 15 minutes of cooldown. This can be similar to your warm-up, but doesn't need to be as demanding or strenuous. Do something you enjoy: walking, treadmill—anything to keep moving. Another great alternative, especially if you're tired, is to focus mostly on just stretching and breathing. Nothing fancy about the stretching—touch your toes, roll your shoulders, just feel where the tension is and try to relax it. Use your breath. Breathe into the stretch. Don't strain. Your workout is over.

Phase One | Tuesday | *Yoga Day*

On Tuesday it's time to back away from the grunt-and-grind of strength training and redirect your body's energies. You need a softer, more fluid form of exercise to rest your stressed muscles and rejuvenate your system. Yoga is perfect for that.

Interestingly, you'll be building lots of new muscle mass on Tuesday, because of the residual effects of Monday's strength workout. Muscle mass doesn't increase as you exercise—it increases during the rest-and-recovery phase following exercise.

Yoga Day isn't just a day of rest, though. It's critically important, because it will add not just to your physical strength, but also to your mental and spiritual strength, which are crucial to fitness. The literal translation of yoga is "to yoke," or "to join"—meaning that yoga is uniquely effective at joining the mind and the body. By dispelling the duality of the mind body separation, yoga empowers both entities tremendously.

Yoga will bring you into yourself. It will increase your awareness of not just the world around you, but also of your own inner world. A recent study showed that yoga was quite effective at helping people lose weight, but this was achieved partly because of yoga's mental effects, rather than its physical effects. In this study, there was an average difference of nineteen pounds of weight loss over several years between people who practiced yoga and people who didn't. The director of the study believed much of this weight loss came simply from people getting more in touch with their bodies, through yoga, and becoming more sensitive to harmful habits, such as overeating.

Yoga does, of course, also have powerful physical effects. It is superb for stretching and strengthening muscles, opening the lungs, increasing flexibility, nurturing the joints, improving posture, and calming the body's nervous system, which results in heightened immunity. As you may remember, even something as simple as *ujjayi* breathing can have profound effects. Be sure to incorporate this breath work into your exercises.

Enjoy your Yoga Day. And remember: Breathe better and feel better. Pleasure can be even more healing than pain.

WARM-UP

Do the usual: Perform any type of light exercise that increases your heart rate by approximately 50 percent. Do 15 minutes.

The 30-Minute Workout

As mentioned in the first workout, this workout was designed to take 30 minutes, but you may not get it all quite done in 30 minutes, or you may finish a little early, and need to repeat some movements to fulfill your 30 minutes.

Target: Your hips.

How-To: Sit as pictured, with your legs in a V position, and push your pelvis and lower back forward. Keep your spine straight, and stretch it out long. Inhale. Then, as you exhale, reach forward toward your toes. Hold that position.

How Long: Hold it for 2 minutes.

The Details:
- ▶ DO: Ease up the exertion on your stretch as you inhale, and push a little farther into the stretch as you exhale.
- ▶ DO: Keep the curve out of your spine as much as possible, to protect your lower back.
- ▶ DO: Bend your knees if you need to, in order to keep from stressing your lower back. This movement is all about the hips, not the back.
- ▶ DON'T: Strain to touch your toes—keep it comfortable.

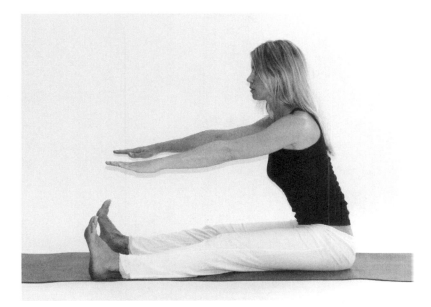

2. BOUND ANGLE POSE

Target: Your inner groin, and your inside thighs.

How-To: Sit with the sides of your feet together, as pictured. Inhale, and stretch your spine upward. Then exhale, as you push forward with your pelvis, lower back, upper body, and arms. Hold that pose.

How Long: Hold it for 2 minutes.

The Details:

▶ DO: Push the outside edges of your feet together for leverage, and then open your feet, as if they were the covers of a book. This unlocks your knees and the backs of your thighs.

▶ DO: Ease up on your stretch during the inhale, and go a little deeper on the exhale.

▶ DON'T: Overstretch. Protect your lower back.

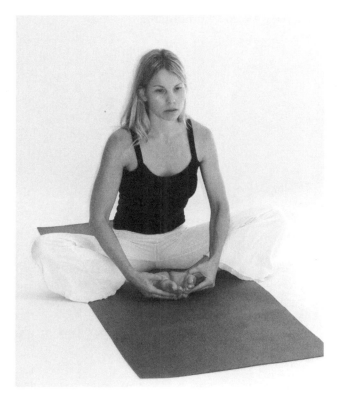

3. HALF-PIGEON POSE

Target: Hips (it opens them).

How-To: Bend your right knee, as pictured, and bring your right heel toward your left hip. Stretch your left leg all the way back behind you, and let your upper body sink down to the floor. Hold this position. Then do the same thing with your other side. If your hip feels stressed, support it somewhat with a folded towel or blanket.

How Long: Hold it for 1½ minutes on each side.

The Details:

▶ DO: Keep the top of the foot that is reaching back flat to the floor, so that you won't twist your knee. This is a hip opener, not a knee twister.

▶ DO: Keep your hips square to the floor.

▶ DON'T: Lengthen through your stretching leg on the inhale. On the exhale, surrender more deeply into the stretch, with your hip a little closer to the ground.

▶ DON'T: Try this pose if you have a knee injury. Instead, do it while lying flat on your back.

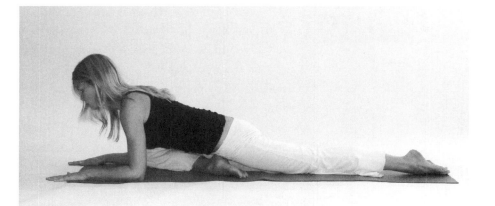

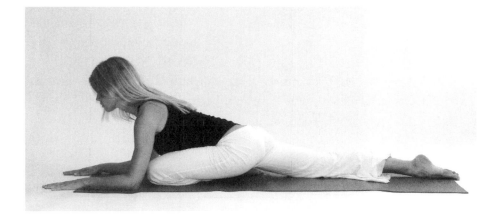

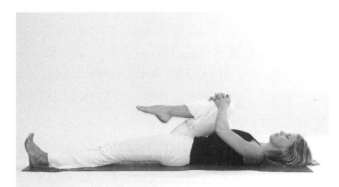

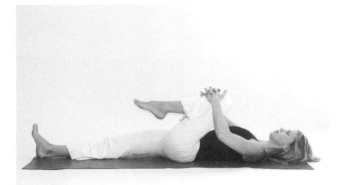

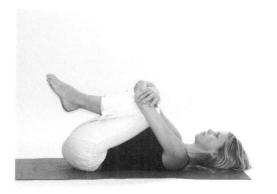

Target: Your abdomen. This posture is especially valuable for expelling gas from and toning the large intestine.

How-To: Lie on your back, as pictured, and bring your right knee toward your chest. Hold it. Then release that knee, and do the same thing with the other knee. Hold it. Then do both knees, and hold that position.

How Long: Hold the 3 postures for 1 minute each, for a total of 3 minutes.

The Details:

▶ DO: Keep your head on the floor, with your chin slightly tucked in, to protect your neck. Resist the temptation to lift your head to watch what you're doing.

▶ DO: Keep the leg that's not bent actively involved, with the toes of that leg pointing up toward the sky.

▶ DO: If you prefer, you can drink a glass of warm water before you do this particular movement, to improve your intestine's peristaltic action.

▶ DO: Squeeze your belly in, and push your lower back into the floor, for extra muscle involvement.

▶ DO: Avoid your rib cage as you pull up your knee, to help put extra pressure on the descending and ascending sections of your large intestine. This movement is especially helpful during cleansing, when your body will be aggressively ridding itself of toxic debris, via the colon.

▶ DON'T: Keep the leg that's on the floor straight and rigid, if you have any type of back problem. Bend it a little, to reduce pressure on your back.

▶ DON'T: Lift your head. That might stress your neck. Keep your head on the floor, with your chin slightly tucked.

5. RECLINING BIG-TOE POSTURE

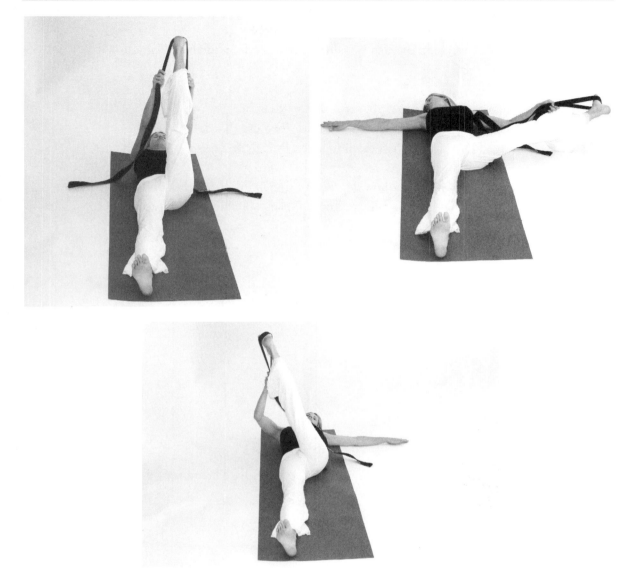

Target: The back of your legs, your hamstring muscles, your hips, and the illiotibial (I.T.) muscle band that runs from your outside thighs to your waist.

How-To: Lying as pictured, bring up your left leg, with a strap (or belt, or long towel) across the ball of your left foot. Pull your left leg back toward your face, with your knee straight. Hold it. Then move your leg to the left, as pictured. For counterbalance, reach out with your right arm, and look to the right. Keep both hips on the floor. Then bring your left leg back to center, and grab the strap with your other hand (your right hand).

(continued on next page)

Bring your head to center. Pull your right leg about 3 inches across the right side of your body, to stretch the outside of your left thigh, and to engage your I.T. muscle band. Then release it, and do the other leg.

How Long: Hold each movement, on each side, for 30 seconds, for a total of 3 minutes.

The Details:
- ▶ DO: Keep your foot flexed, and bring your toes toward your face.
- ▶ DO: Keep the opposite leg active and strong, with that foot also flexed.
- ▶ DO: Ease up on the inhale, and exert yourself more on the exhale.
- ▶ DON'T: Lift the hips off the floor.
- ▶ DON'T: Overstretch. This isn't about how far you can stretch. It's about the subtle movements.
- ▶ DON'T: Lift your head. That might strain your neck. Keep your chin slightly tucked.

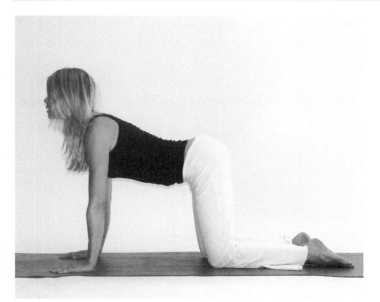

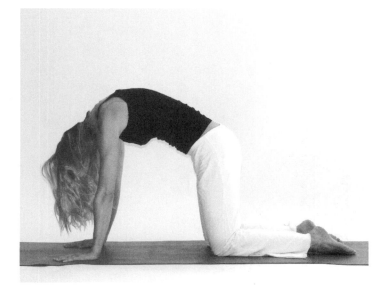

Target: Your abdomen. Your back. This posture creates flexibility and strength in both. It also loosens the spine and improves nervous system function.

How-To: Get on all fours, as pictured and inhale as you arch your back. Keep head up, inhale, and lower your head down as you tuck your chin to your neck. Pull your belly up—and bring your tailbone down—as you round your back, as if you were a cat stretching.

How Many: Do 5 reps.

The Details:

▶ DC: Keep your knees directly in line with your hips, and hands with shoulders.
▶ DC: Keep your hands and knees shoulder-width apart, to achieve complete balance.
▶ DON'T: Lock your elbows, even though your arms are straight.
▶ DON'T: Overstretch. This is meant to strengthen the spine, not heighten flexibility.

7. DOWNWARD DOG POSE

Target: This strengthens and lengthens the back of your entire body, including the backs of your legs. It also strengthens your shoulders, arms, and wrists. In addition, it increases circulation to your brain, and stimulates endocrine function.

How-To: Stay on all fours, and inhale. Then exhale, and push your hips up high into an inverted V shape. Hold it.

How Long: Hold it for 2 minutes.

The Details:
- ▶ DO: Push strongly with your arms, with your elbows in.
- ▶ DO: Relax your face and neck, with your chin pulled in, in order to keep your spine stretched and long. Keep your ears in line with your biceps.
- ▶ DO: Use your imagination, visualizing yourself doing a perfect version of the inverted V posture.
- ▶ DO: Reach your heels to the ground, and bend your knees, if the posture becomes too difficult.
- ▶ DON'T: Allow your inner thighs to roll out.

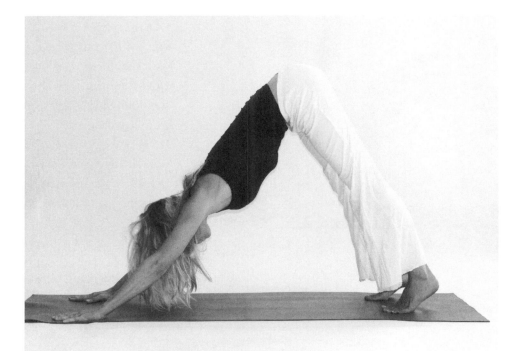

8. CHILD'S POSE

Target: This stretches your arms and the back of your body, and opens up your chest and shoulders. It relaxes and restores the energy system. It's the beginning of your cooldown.

How-To: Coming out of the Downward Dog Pose, inhale, then exhale, and bend your knees toward the floor. Bring your tailbone back, and down, toward your heels, as pictured. Keep your arms stretched ahead of you, with your forehead resting on the floor. Hold it.

How Long: Hold it for 2 minutes.

The Details:
▶ DO: Keep your elbows off the floor.
▶ DON'T: Lift your head.

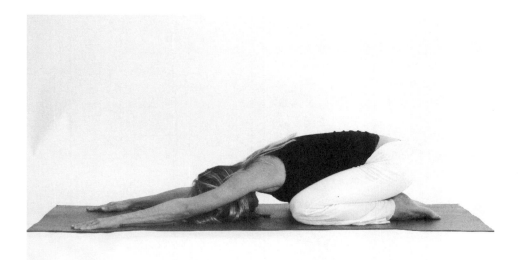

9. SPINE TWIST

Target: The spinal column. This movement helps create space between your spine's vertebrae, and thereby increases the nerve supply to your internal organs, including your heart, lungs, spleen, and kidneys.

How-To: Sitting as pictured, bring up your right knee, and cross it over your left thigh. Sit up tall, and stretch your left arm up and over your right knee. For support, keep your right hand behind you. On the inhale, stretch up through your spine, to create vertebral space. On the exhale, twist your upper body to the right, as you look to the right. Hold it. Then repeat the move on the other side.

How Long: Hold it for 30 seconds on each side.

The Details:

▶ DO: Bend the arm that's behind you as you twist, to allow for greater opening of the front of your body.
▶ DO: Ease up on the inhale breath, and twist a little deeper on the exhale breath on each side.
▶ DON'T: Overstretch your neck, by looking too far back. Allow your head to follow your body.

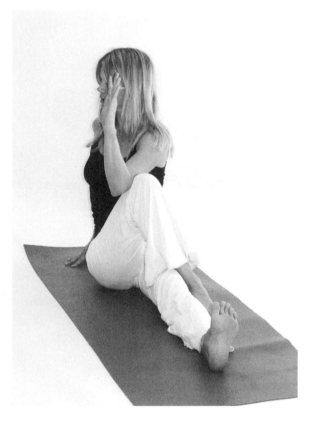

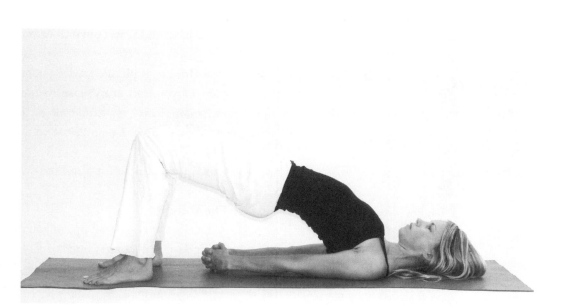

Target: This opens the front of your body, and releases heat. It can also help release pent-up emotions.

How-To: Lie as pictured, with your feet hip-width apart, your knees bent, and your feet flat. Your head should be on the floor, with your chin slightly tucked. Inhale, then exhale as you raise your hips up. Interlace your fingers under your hips. Squeeze your shoulder blades together, to release your lower back. At the conclusion, release your body, then your arms, roll to your right into a fetal position, and take a moment to relax before sitting up.

How Long: Hold it for 2 minutes.

The Details:
▶ DO: Stay with your breath. Use it to help do the work.
▶ DON'T: Look sideways. You might stress your neck.

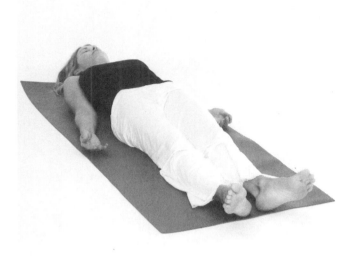

Target: Your mind and emotions. This promotes inner peace and physical relaxation.

How-To: Lie as pictured, with your legs in front of you and arms close to the body with palms facing up, head to floor, slightly tucked, chin to chest, and close your eyes.

How Long: Hold it for 5 minutes.

The Details:

► DO: Bring your head up, so you can see if you're in a straight line.
► DO: Relax your face, neck, and shoulders, and feel the relaxation spread down your body.
► DO: Raise your legs up against a wall, if you're feeling tense from cleansing. This will increase circulation to your brain, and help you relax and focus.
► DO: Say a prayer of thanks at the end.
► DON'T: Leave your eyes open. Close them. Surrender to your breath. Relax your jaw, and allow tension to leave your body.
► DON'T: Let troubling thoughts take over your mind. Acknowledge them, and let go.
► DON'T: Hold in tension. Let it go.

COOLDOWN

Your cooldown is the Corpse Pose. As you near the end of your workout, focus on what you've achieved.

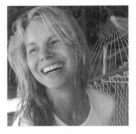

Irma Joujon-Roche, who helped develop your yoga workout, is a multifaceted expert on health, nutrition, and fitness, and has studied natural modalities on three continents.

Reared and educated in Europe, she moved to Australia in the 1980s, where she managed a chain of gymnasiums, and studied aerobics, gymnastics, and aquatics.

Following a successful entrepreneurship in the fashion industry, she moved to California to attend the American University of Complementary Medicine. There she studied nutrition, traditional Chinese medicine, and acupuncture, and learned to apply the Five Element Theory and the Meridian System to traditional fitness and health techniques. She eventually began to specialize in yoga, under the mentorship of a yoga master.

She currently works with her husband, Gregory Joujon-Roche, as his primary consultant on the nutritional programs of various stars, and also as a consultant on yoga. She is also the director of the Six Essentials line of nutritional supplements, which are used by many holistic fitness clients.

Phase One | **Wednesday** | *Pilates Day*

Now we focus on the area of your body that you probably have the biggest problem with: your core, including your abdominal muscles, butt, hips, thighs, and belly. Those are the main trouble spots for most people.

Pilates directly addresses this core area, which is called the powerhouse in Pilates terminology. Because so many people have problems with this area, Pilates has enjoyed huge success over the past few years.

Pilates was created in the early 1900s by a German immigrant named Joseph Pilates, who was seeking a highly systematized, orderly approach to fitness. He came to believe that fitness starts in the powerhouse, and emanates outward from there.

Because Pilates exercises are precise, they require focus, concentration, and attention to detail—qualities that I believe are the keys to all avenues of high-level fitness.

When mental focus is applied to exercises aimed at the powerhouse, the abdomen and torso become the center of the body's strength, and enable the body to avoid injuries and trauma in its extremities.

A body trained with Pilates tends to acquire these attributes:

- A taut, well-toned abdomen
- A taller, lengthened posture
- Lean, sinewy leg muscles
- Firm buttocks
- A resistance to injury
- Gracefulness

Although some Pilates work requires equipment, the Pilates work you will do in this program is floor-based mat work, which many people consider the most valuable form of Pilates exercise. This mat work is challenging, but it really pays off. Your Pilates mat work is derived from forty mat exercises created by Joseph Pilates. They are performed as you lie on your back, front, or sides, or as you sit on the floor. These exercises consist of movements that target muscles deep in your abdominal and spinal areas.

They are not designed as aerobic exercises, but focus instead upon strength, toning, flexibility, and coordination.

Once you get into the swing of Pilates, you'll really start to notice the difference in your body.

Neutral Position Used in All Pilates Exercises

The Neutral Position is one where the core (the powerhouse) is constantly engaged by pulling in the belly button, positioning your heels in and your toes out, all while zipping up the inner thighs and squeezing the butt. Also essential to maintaining the Neutral Position is keeping the tailbone centered (not sticking out or too far tucked under).

The other important component is breath. We want to teach our bodies how to consciously take in more oxygen while moving our muscles. The rule of thumb in practicing Pilates is to breathe opposite to the motion. Instead of exhaling as the muscle engages the most (e.g., at the top of a sit-up), one inhales on the effort and exhales on the release. With practice you will find a profound increase in energy while complementing the other workouts.

WARM-UP

Do the usual 15 minutes. Get your heart going. Have fun. Connect with your self.

Your 30-Minute Workout

As before, if you finish before 30 minutes, do some repeats.

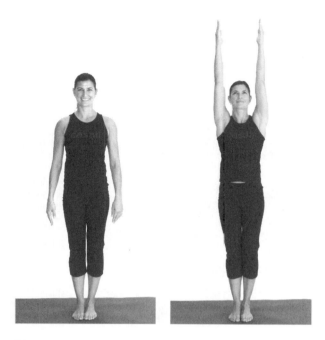

Target: Your core—or, in Pilates terminology, your powerhouse. Virtually all of these Pilates mat exercises target the powerhouse: all the muscles between the ribs and hips—particularly the abs, the lower back, and the butt.

How-To: Start by standing in Neutral Position, as pictured, and explained at the beginning of this segment. Bring your arms overhead, tuck your chin in to your chest, then bring them down slowly. Visualize stretching your spine, one vertebra at a time, until your hands touch the floor. Then slowly come back up, opening your hamstrings and spine.

How Many: 10 reps

The Details:

▶ DO: Exhale and stretch overhead at the end.

▶ DO: Tuck in your chin as you go down toward the floor.

▶ DON'T: Push your belly out. Pull it up toward your heart, to help you stay connected to your powerhouse.

▶ DON'T: Rush it. Take your time. If you hurry, you'll disengage from your powerhouse.

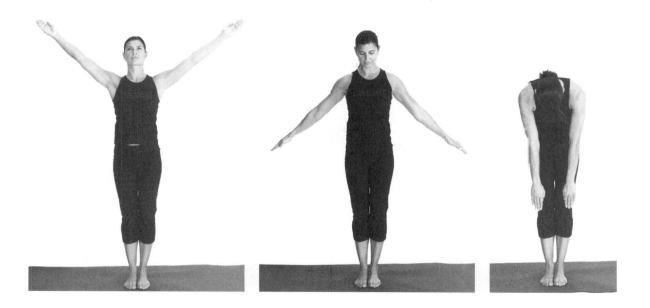

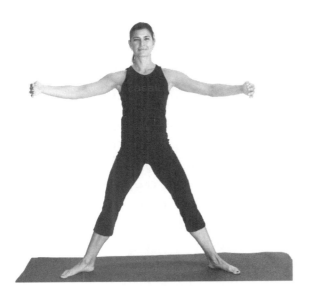

Target: Your legs. Primarily, your inner thighs.

How-To: Stand with your legs wide and your toes turned out, as pictured. Squat down, and come back up. As you squat, keep your powerhouse engaged: Tighten it, and stay conscious of it.

How Many: 3 sets of 10 reps

The Details:
▶ DO: Breathe with a conscious, regular flow.
▶ DON'T: Lean forward. That could strain your hips.
▶ DON'T: Slide your knee over your toe—keep it over the heel. This will help protect your knees.

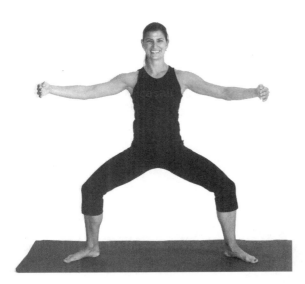

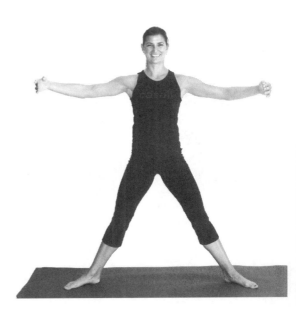

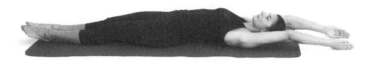

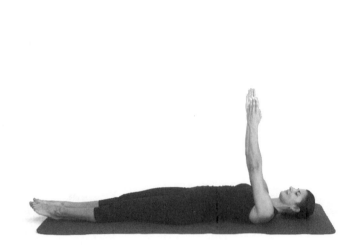

Target: The powerhouse—the abs, back, butt, and inner thighs.

How-To: Lie as pictured, and engage your powerhouse. Keep your ribs soft, and slowly roll up from the mat, one vertebra at a time, relying on only the strength of your abs, rather than momentum. Then slowly return to first position, as pictured.

How Many: 10 reps

The Details:

- ▶ DO: Inhale on the exertion, and exhale on the release.
- ▶ DO: Go slowly. Keep the work in your muscles.
- ▶ DO: Visualize your vertebrae opening and separating. This is all about massaging the spine open, and working the muscles that are closest to the spine.
- ▶ DON'T: Check out, and release the muscles of the inner thigh. Stay connected.
- ▶ DON'T: Hold your breath. As always, in Pilates, inhale on the effort and exhale on the release.
- ▶ DON'T: Shrug your shoulders. That pulls effort away from the powerhouse, and it can also hurt your neck.

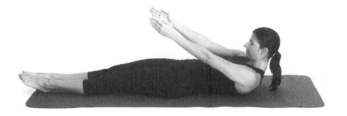

(continued on next page)

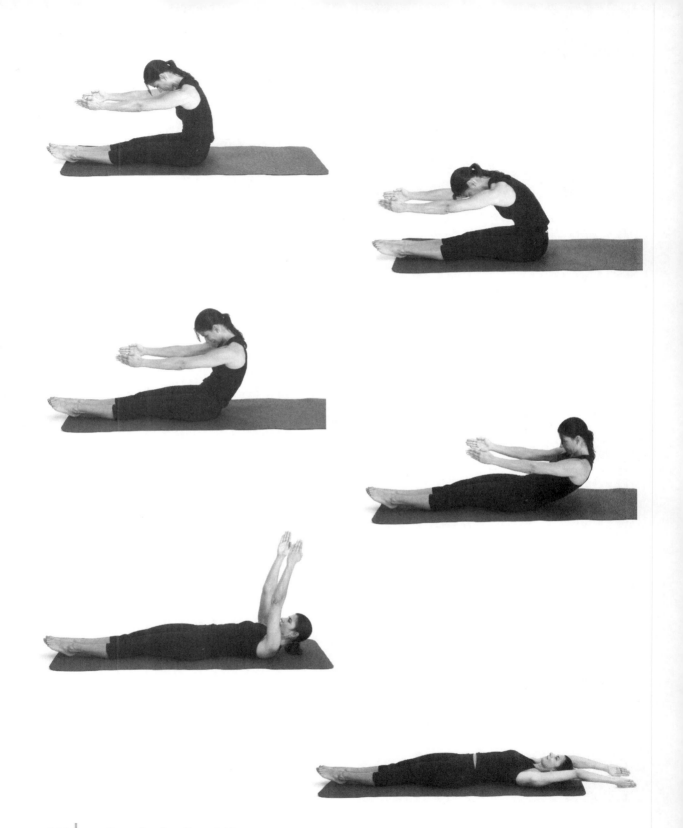

4. THE HUNDREDS

Target: The entire powerhouse. Also, your heart rate—this is aerobically strenuous.

How-To: Lie on your back, on a mat or soft surface, in a "tabletop" position, as pictured, with your knees over your hips, and your feet pointed. Then raise your chest and head up, look over your knees, and hold the position. As you do it, extend your arms along your thighs, and move them rhythmically, as if you were paddling water. Keep moving them throughout the exercise.

How Long: Hold it for 5 counts and 5 paddles on every inhale, and also on every exhale.

How Many: 10 reps

The Details:
▶ DO: Keep your chest raised. If you're too low, the exercise loses its impact. Think of your spine as having a C shape.
▶ DON'T: Lean your head back. That could strain your neck and vertebrae.
▶ DON'T: Pull your knees too far in. You might strain your hip flexors, and you'll make the exercise lazy.

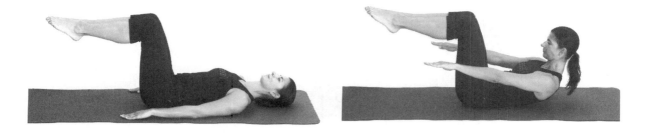

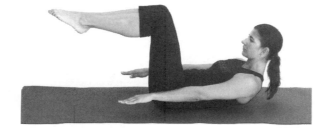

5. SINGLE-LEG STRETCHES

Target: The powerhouse and also the legs.

How-To: Lie on your back and bring both knees to your chest, as you simultaneously lift your chest, and also chin, up toward your knees. Engage your powerhouse. Then extend one leg, and keep the other bent, as pictured. Do 10 quick pulls, or "pulses," on each leg—alternating legs—while you keep your upper body stable. Next, add an upper-body twist to the exercise. To do this, put your hands behind your head, and touch one of your knees with your opposite elbow, as pictured. This time, don't do the quick pulses. Do 10 touches to each knee.

How Many: 10 pulses on each leg, and 10 knee-touches on each leg

The Details:
- ▶ DO: Keep your hips stable.
- ▶ DON'T: Collapse your legs. Keep them up at almost 90-degree angles.
- ▶ DON'T: Drop your shoulders. That can hurt, and it can keep you from getting the proper workout.

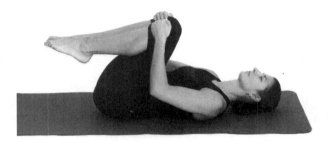

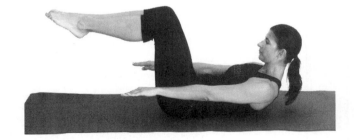

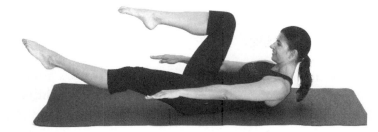

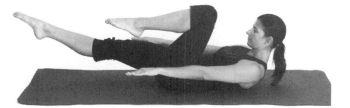

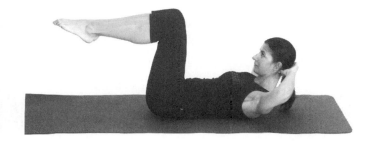

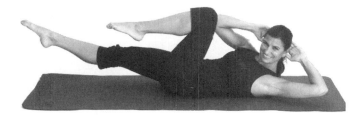

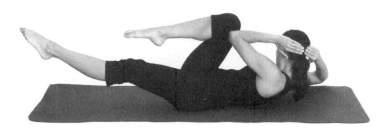

6. SINGLE STRAIGHT-LEG STRETCHES

The Target: The powerhouse (primarily your abs, back, and inner thighs).

How-To: Get in the same position as Single-Leg Stretch. Now, though, pulse your legs like scissors, as pictured, with one leg straight up and the other hovering just over the mat. Do 10 pulses. Then grab one of your calf muscles with your opposite hand—while you extend the other arm overhead, as pictured— and twist your torso. Hold your calf throughout the twist. Do 10 twists touching one knee to the opposite elbow. Then change legs, and do 10 more.

How Many: 10 pulses, 10 twists on each side

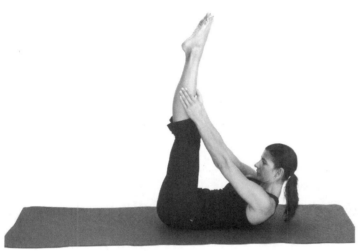

The Details:
- ► DO: Move slowly. That's the way to fully engage each muscle.
- ► DON'T: Sway your back. It takes the effort away from where it belongs.
- ► DON'T: Rely on your arms. Make your powerhouse do the work.

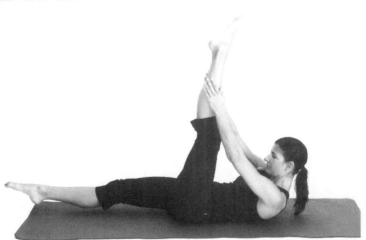

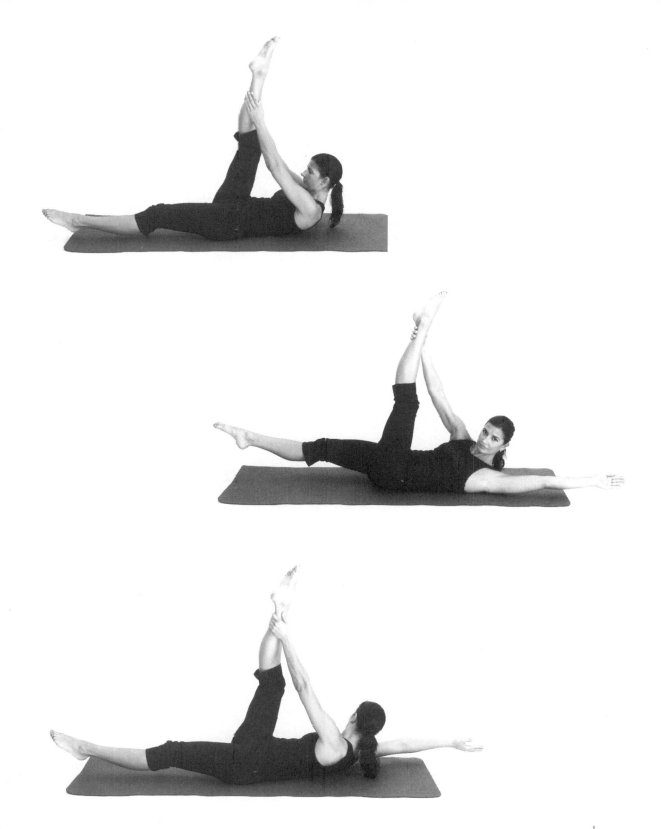

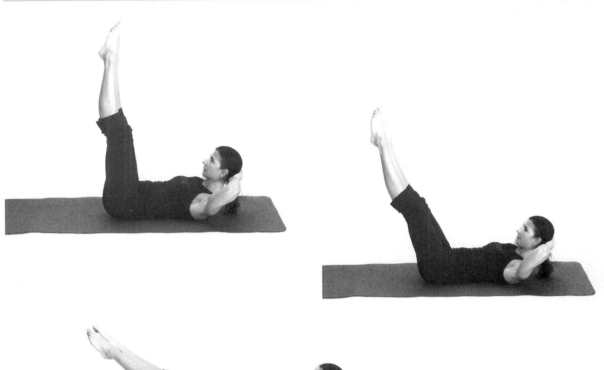

Target: The lower abs, mostly, but also the entire powerhouse.

How-To: Lift both legs straight up in the air, as pictured. Then bring them slowly down, under control, and lift them again, using your abs.

How Many: 10 reps

The Details:
- ▶ DO: Stay connected to your lower abs. Live in your abs. Own them.
- ▶ DO: Keep your lower back against the floor, to help you stay in touch with your powerhouse.
- ▶ DON'T: Push your abs out. That decreases the work.
- ▶ DON'T: Drop your shoulders.

8. ROLLING LIKE A BALL

Target: Your powerhouse.

How-To: Sit at the edge of a mat, as pictured, with your knees pulled into your chest, your hands to your ankles, and your elbows pulled into your sides. Then slowly arch (or round) your back, as you assume the rounded shape of a ball. Next, roll back on the floor, engaging your powerhouse, and roll back up again to a sitting position, without letting your feet touch the floor.

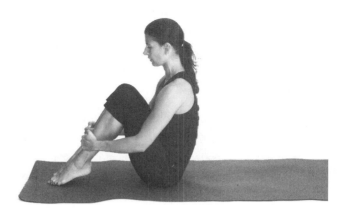

How Many: 10 reps

The Details:

▶ DO: Keep your chin tucked, to protect your neck.

▶ DO: Keep your knees tight to your body.

▶ DON'T: Straighten your back while you're rolling. That can injure it. Keep it rounded.

▶ DON'T: Check out. Stay in your vertebrae.

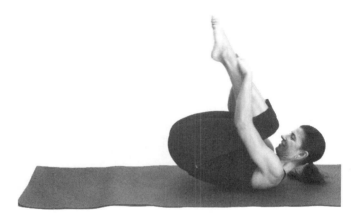

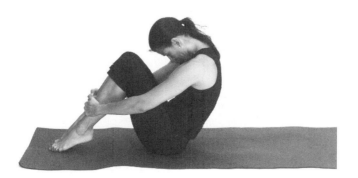

(continued on next page)

COOLDOWN

Try to do about 15 minutes of mild movement. Get some fresh air! Catch your breath. Feel the energy flow.

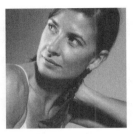

Tanja Djelevic, who helped develop your Pilates workout, was recently named one of "The Top 100 Trainers in America" by *Men's Journal.* She trains the A-list of Hollywood stars, including Jennifer Garner, Uma Thurman, and Matt Dillon. A former track and field star in her native Sweden, she holds a master's degree in sports psychology, and specializes in Pilates, dance, kinesiology, and stress management. She is the fitness columnist for the Swedish edition of *Cosmopolitan* magazine, and directs fitness programs at Paramount Pictures, Gold's Gym, and Hollywood's Crunch Fitness. She began her career as a dancer in theater, and attended the prestigious Swedish Academy of Fitness Education. Her workout programs are famous in the Los Angeles area for their ability to evoke physical energy and emotional inspiration.

Phase One | **Thursday** | *Martial Arts Day*

Today's the day to have some fun, and play action hero. Your martial arts workout is going to feel great, and it's going to relieve stress you didn't even know you had. And, it's also going to burn calories like nothing else! Thirty minutes of martial arts can oxidize almost a quarter-pound of body fat. You don't get that kind of calorie burn on a treadmill.

All martial arts are fighting systems, generally used by people who are unarmed—although sometimes handheld weapons, such as swords, are used. There are many styles of martial arts—including karate, tae kwon do, judo, and kung fu—most of which were developed long ago in Asia. All forms of martial arts are intended to enable people to physically defend themselves from others, or to defeat others. Because martial arts have this serious purpose, they have been refined throughout the ages to be exceedingly efficient in their employment of the human body's power. There are no wasted movements in martial arts, so this form of physical movement requires focus, mindfulness, and attention to detail. Therefore, the physical actions of martial arts have a powerful impact upon the body. It's just about impossible to practice martial arts without getting into great shape.

Furthermore, this fitness will be attained throughout the body, because physical combat, by its very nature, demands the full use of the body.

Although the styles of martial arts vary widely, most martial arts revolve around two essential movements: punches and kicks. You might think that this means using just your arms, or just your legs, but once you try these movements, you'll see that they require muscle activity throughout the body.

The fighting activities in martial arts will help you to express your stress: You can't do a dynamic kick or punch without involving your emotions. When you've had a hard day, nothing feels better than physicalizing your frustration, and getting rid of it.

Similarly to my approach to the other exercise disciplines, such as Pilates or yoga, no experience is required. You don't need to be an expert. These workouts have all been customized for simplicity, synergy . . . and fun!

So get going, have a blast, and take note of how much better you feel at the end of this workout.

WARM-UP

Try a more strenuous form of warm-up: jumping rope. Try to do about 5 minutes, taking breaks when necessary. If you don't enjoy it, do another challenging form of warm-up, such as jogging, or walking uphill.

Your 30-Minute Workout

If you finish early, keep going until 30 minutes have elapsed.

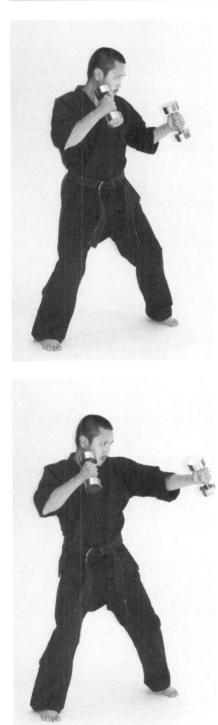

Target: Your entire torso, except for the pectoral muscles in your chest. Mostly, though, this targets your arms, shoulders, back, abs, and obliques.

How-To: Begin in a standard boxing stance, as pictured, with weights in your hands—no less than 2 pounds each. Imagine that you're standing on a clock, and face 12 o'clock, with your feet at 11 and 5, as pictured. Your toes should be at 45-degree angles. Keep your knees soft, and your weight equally distributed. Now you're ready for a series of three different kinds of punches: (A) jab, (B) jab-cross combination, and (C) jab-cross-hook combination.

Caution: Because you have weights in your hand, you'll need to focus on grace and control. Jerky, flailing movements invite unnecessary strain.

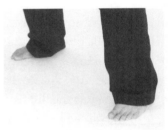

A. JAB

How-To: If you're right-handed, your left side should be forward, facing your imaginary opponent. Then punch at a slow to medium pace with your left hand, while holding the weight. Go almost, but not quite, to a full extension of your arm. Keep your other hand, also holding a weight, up near your cheek or ear, as if ready to defend yourself.

How Many: Do 15 reps, or punches, on each side.

The Details:

▶ DO: Pick the right amount of weight—one that's not too heavy.

▶ DO: Aim at the height of your own head. If you prefer, you can do this in front of a mirror, and aim toward your head.

▶ DO: Keep your arm jabbing straight ahead.

▶ DO: Keep your knees relaxed.

▶ DON'T: Sacrifice your form by using a weight that's too heavy. You'll decrease the value of the martial arts workout.

▶ DON'T: Hyperextend your arm. You can strain your elbow.

B. JAB-CROSS COMBINATION

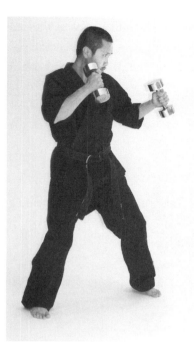

How-To: Do a jab, followed immediately by a cross with the other hand. A cross is a punch with the rear hand that crosses over your body to get to the opponent's body, as pictured. It's a powerful punch, similar to swinging a baseball bat hard enough to hit a home run. Your right foot pivots, to bring your whole body into it. Your lower body should turn all the way around, until your hips are facing the front.

How Many: Do 15 reps of the whole combination on each side.

The Details:

▶ DO: Make sure you turn your hips.
▶ DO: Pivot on the ball of your foot, to keep your legs in the exercise.
▶ DO: Make sure you're jabbing in a straight line.
▶ DON'T: Overextend. Neither punch should extend the arm all the way.

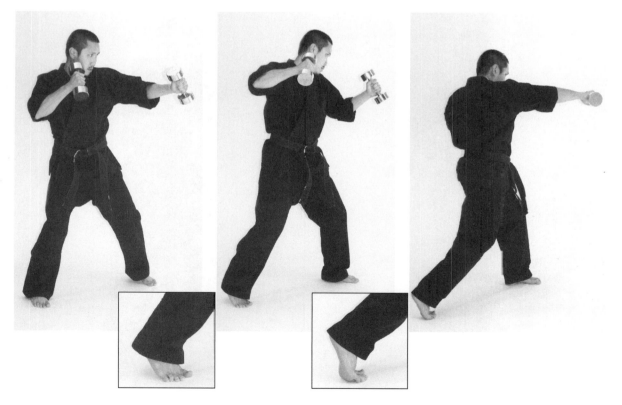

C. JAB-CROSS-HOOK COMBINATION

How-To: With your same side still forward, throw the jab-cross combination, and add a hook at the end of it. A hook is an oval-shaped punch that is intended to avoid your opponent's arms, and strike the opponent on the side of the head. Throw it with your lead hand, as pictured. End the combination back in the guard position, with both hands up.

How Many: Do 15 reps with one hand leading, then turn to the other side and do 15 more with the other hand leading.

The Details:

▶ DO: Stay in control—especially since you have weights in your hands. Take care to keep from striking yourself with the weights.
▶ DON'T: Make the oval of the cross too wide—that can hurt your shoulder.

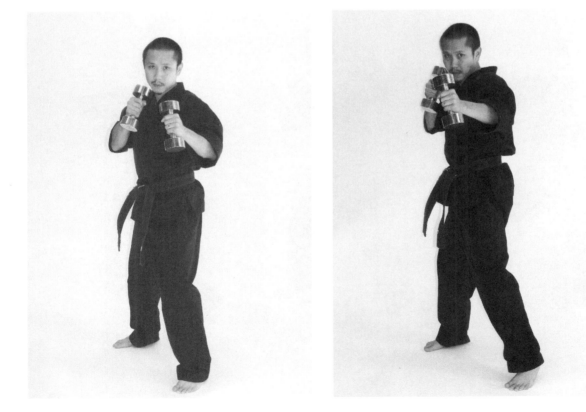

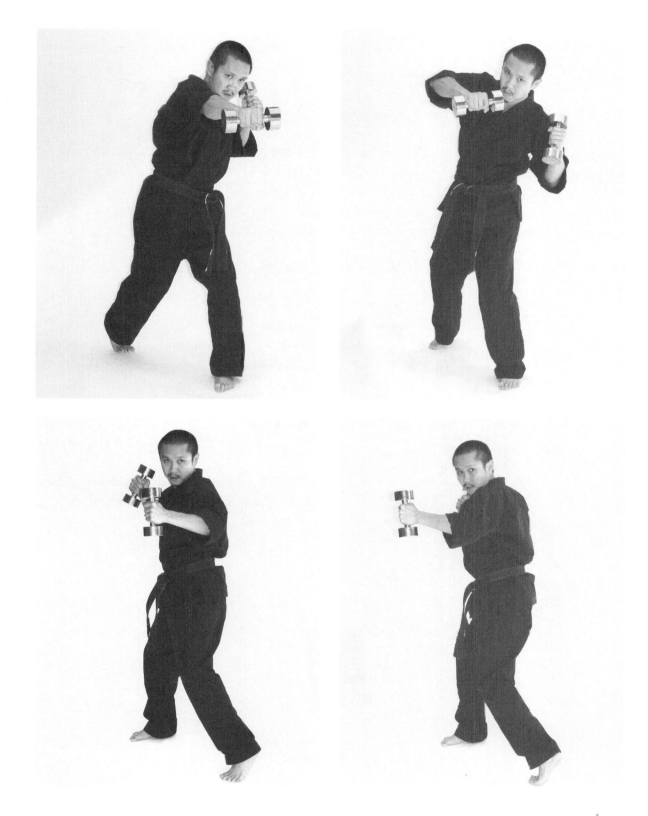

2. KICKS

The only kick in Phase One is the classic roundhouse kick.

Target: Your obliques, abs, and the entire leg, except for the calves.

How-To: Hold on to the back of a chair, or anything else that will help support you, such as a wall or table. Lift your right knee to a V position, as pictured. Then slowly extend your leg, as pictured, and drop it. Do this 20 times slowly, then do the same move 20 times quickly. On the very last of the quick kicks, hold your leg out, as high as possible, and then pulse it quickly upward twenty times, bringing it up about 3 to 5 inches each time. Then switch sides, and do the other leg.

How Many: Do 3 sets with each leg. That consists of 20 slow lifts, 20 fast lifts, and 20 pulses, for each leg, 3 different times.

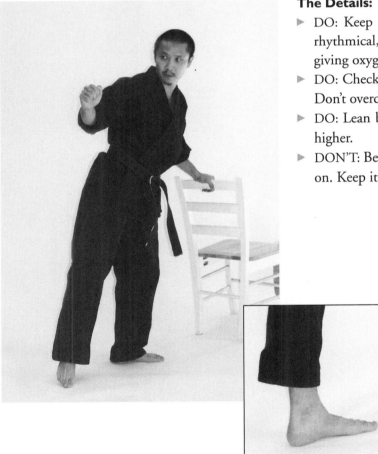

The Details:

▶ DO: Keep your breath in it. It helps you stay rhythmical, and feeds your muscles with energy-giving oxygen.
▶ DO: Check in with your body when you finish. Don't overdo it.
▶ DO: Lean back a little if you want to kick even higher.
▶ DON'T: Bend the knee of the leg you're standing on. Keep it locked without hyperextending.

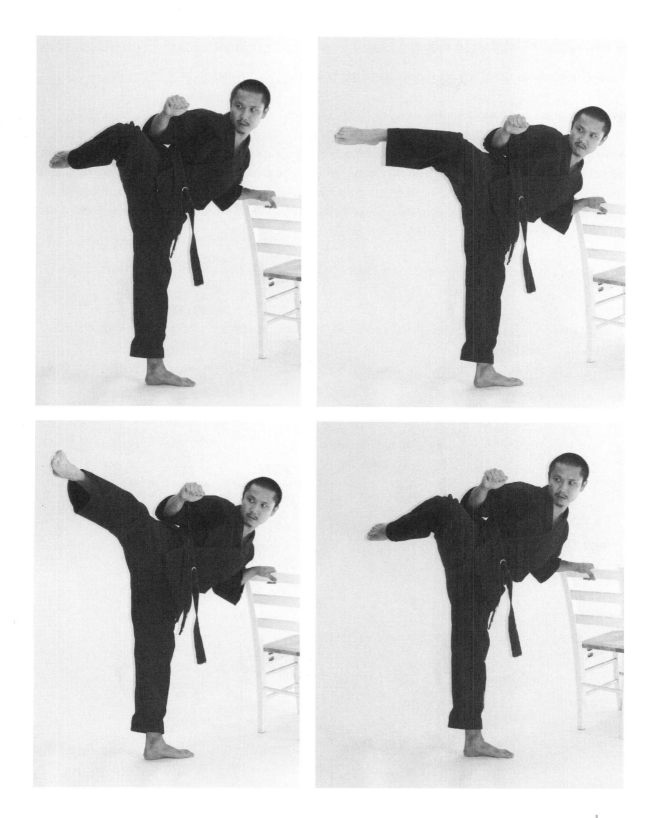

3. THAI KNEE-ABS

In Thai kickboxing, the knees are thrown as weapons, in movements that are similar to this.

Target: Your abs and your obliques.

How-To: Lie on your back, with your knees bent and slightly spread, almost as if you are an expectant mother in a birthing position. Then do two "concentrated crunches." That means your abs are very tight and engaged as you do a crunch. Then quickly cross your right elbow to your left knee, as pictured. To do this, bring your chest up and your knee up at the same time. Do it 10 times, then switch to the other elbow and knee.

How Many: Do 3 sets of 10 reps, with each knee.

The Details:

▶ DO: Contract your stomach on the concentrated crunches, expelling your breath in a rigorous "huh" sound.

▶ DON'T: Check out. Stay focused on your abs. Keep the tension in them.

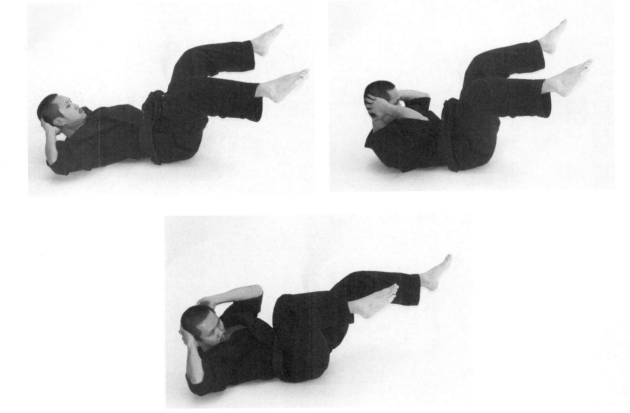

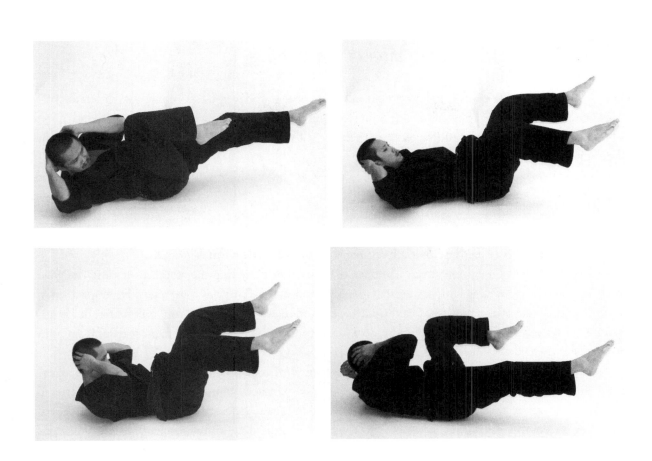

COOLDOWN

Martial arts is one of your more challenging workouts, so you'll probably look forward to the cooldown. Fill your cooldown time with whatever serves you best: stretching, breathing, and listening to your body. Your body always knows what it wants. You just have to learn to listen.

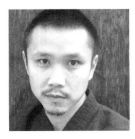

Steven Ho, who designed the martial arts workout, is one of the most sought-after martial arts trainers and choreographers in Hollywood. Shortly after high school, Ho was recruited into the film business by action icon Jet Li, and soon began a Hollywood career by portraying Donatello in the hit films *Teenage Mutant Ninja Turtles II* and *III*. With over fifteen years of stunt and film experience, Ho specializes in getting actors "film ready" in a short period of time. Among others, his students include Brad Pitt, Leonardo DiCaprio, Tobey Maguire, and James Franco.

Phase One | **Friday** | *Core Interval Training Day*

This is the last day of the week, so let's close it out with a bang! Today you'll combine two different types of exercise—core training, plus interval training—which become core interval training.

Core training is similar to Pilates work, because it focuses on the body's core, or powerhouse: the abdomen and torso.

Interval training consists of intervals of aerobic exercise mixed in with the strength work of core training.

Put the two together, and you've got the best of both worlds: the fat-burning power of aerobic exercise, combined with the muscle-building power of strength work. Furthermore, the strength work is focused on the body's core, because that's the primary area of concern for most people.

Core training is aimed not just at whittling the waist and flattening the stomach. It's also designed to strengthen the stabilizing muscles around the hips and pelvis. This has a very positive impact upon posture, and upon correct alignment of the entire skeleton. It not only makes you look better, but is important for preventing injuries. People who do a lot of core work often experience great relief from joint problems in their neck, knees, back, and pelvis.

When the strength work of core training is combined with aerobic interval work, you get a synergistic effect. The added muscle mass from the strength work makes your body burn more calories, and the aerobic exertion of the interval work shoots oxygen and nutrients straight into muscle tissue. In addition, the strength work makes the aerobic work easier, by providing more muscle to do the work, and the aerobic work gives you more stamina for the strength work.

Tomorrow is a day off, so really get into it today. Earn it!

WARM-UP

Cardio Warm-up: Take a brisk walk, jog, or bike ride—anything to get your heart rate and your body temperature up. Go for about 5–10 minutes.

Your 30-Minute Workout

Don't rush it. Use the whole 30 minutes. Core work is all about being in your body—not hurrying around in mindless movement.

3-PART KICK SEQUENCE

1. ON YOUR BACK: This warms your hamstrings, hips, and lower back, while engaging your abs. Lie on your back with your arms at your sides, palms down, and your legs extended. Kick your right leg up toward the ceiling 10 times, then your left leg. After that, bring your arms to the sides, and kick your right leg across your body toward your left hand 10 times. Then kick your left leg toward your right hand 10 times. Take a moment, and let your back settle by taking a big breath, and relaxing.

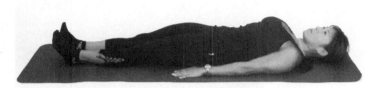

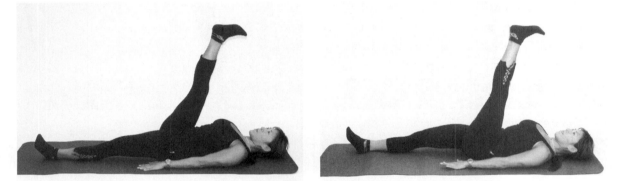

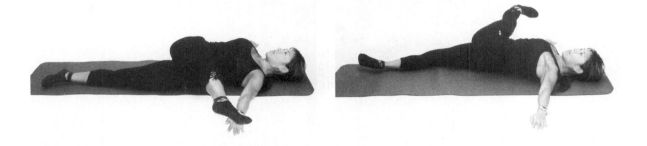

2. STANDING FRONT TO BACK: Stand with your feet together—beside a wall, or something else to hold on to. Kick your outside leg 10 times from front to back. Keep the leg straight as you kick to the front, and bend your knee as you kick to the back, as pictured. Then, turn to the other side, and kick the other leg, front to back, 10 times. Keep your torso upright throughout the exercise.

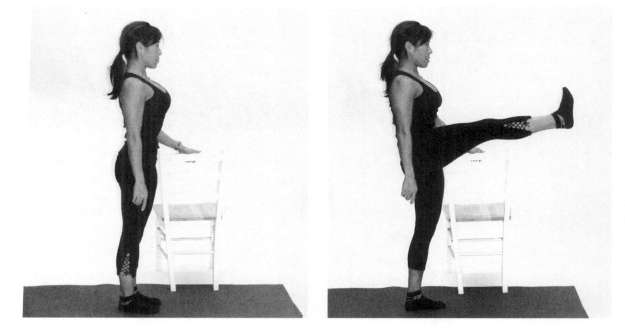

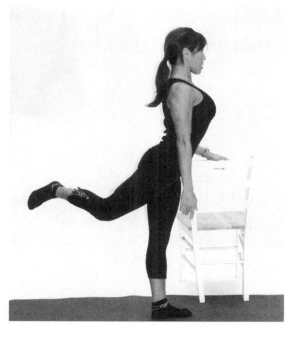

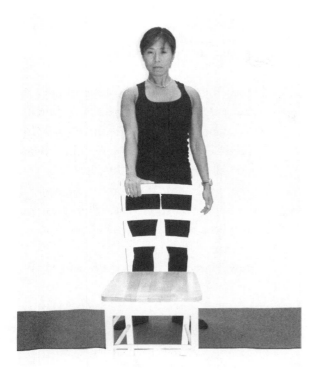

3. STANDING SIDE TO SIDE: Stand facing a wall, or something else to hold on to, with your toes and knees turned outward. Brace yourself with your right hand, and swing your right leg across the front of your body. Then swing it out to the side, back and forth, like a pendulum. Do it 10 times. Switch to the other side, and do 10 more. Keep your torso upright throughout the exercise.

The Details:

▶ DO: Keep good posture.

▶ DO: Keep your abdominals engaged.

▶ DO: Keep your toes pointing toward the ceiling as you kick.

▶ DON'T: Try to kick too hard or high.

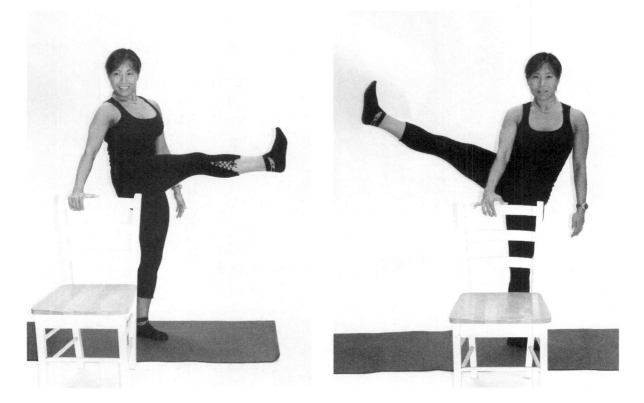

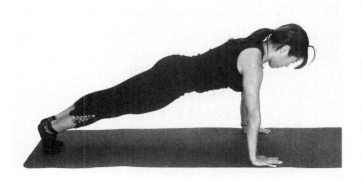

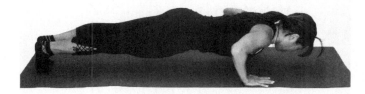

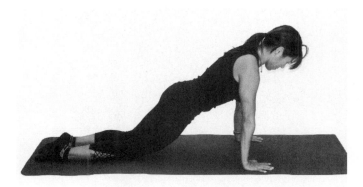

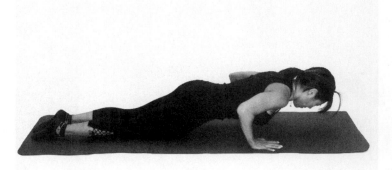

Target: Your upper body and abs.

How-To: Get into a prone position, on your toes (or on your knees, as pictured). Place your hands at least shoulder-width apart—even with your chest line. Bend your elbows to about 90 degrees as you lower your chest and body evenly toward the floor. Straighten your elbows as you push back up to your starting position.

How Many: 15 reps—or do it until you experience muscle fatigue.

The Details:
- DO: Focus on engaging your chest muscles, as you push up.
- DO: Keep your abs tight and hips level.
- DO: Use slow and controlled movements.
- DON'T: Lock your elbows.
- DON'T: Let your hips sag.
- DON'T: Arch your lower back.
- DON'T: Hold your breath. Exhale as you push up.

3. STATIONARY CARDIO INTERVAL

Target: Your heart rate. This should get your heart rate up to about 70 percent of your maximum.

How-To: Do any movement—in place—that you can sustain at a moderately intense pace. This could include doing jumping jacks, jumping rope, or doing high knee lifts.

How Long: 1 minute, 3 times, with short rests in between, for a total of 3 minutes

The Details:
- ▶ DO: Pace yourself to maintain the same intensity throughout the entire minute.
- ▶ DO: Keep good posture while moving.

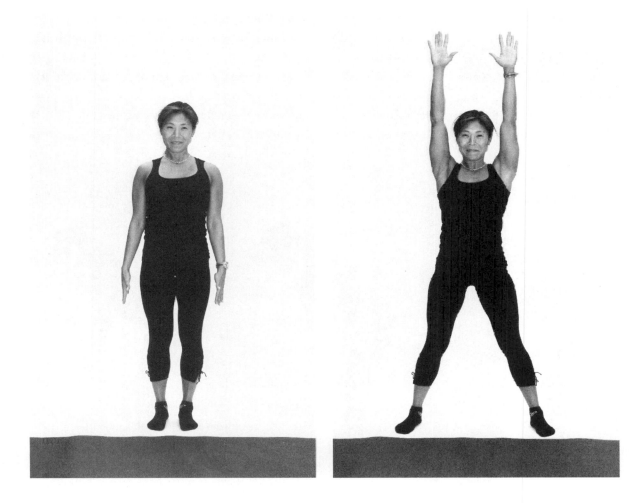

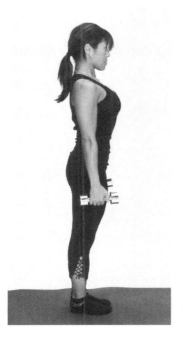

Target: Your upper back, shoulders, and abs.

How-To: Holding on to dumbbells (men: 12–20 pounds; women: 5–10 pounds), stand with your feet close together. Hinge forward at your hips, as pictured. Pull your elbows toward the ceiling, as pictured, while you squeeze your back muscles and rear shoulder muscles.

How Many: 10 to 20

The Details:

▶ DO: Keep your abs engaged, to support your back and to help keep it flat.
▶ DO: Visualize squeezing your shoulder blades together, as you pull your elbows toward the ceiling.
▶ DO: Extend your chest bone forward, toward the top of your head. This helps keep your spine long.
▶ DON'T: Lock your knees. Hinge them enough to feel a nice stretch in your hamstrings.
▶ DON'T: Look up. Keep your eyes focused on one point on the floor. This keeps your neck flat.
▶ DON'T: Let your upper body lift out of the hinge as you row. Stay flat.

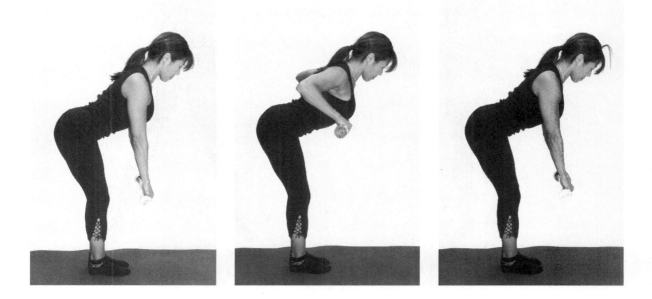

5. LATERAL-SHUFFLE CARDIO INTERVAL

Target: Your heart rate, and the muscles that control lateral (side to side) movement. You don't move only front to back in daily life, but also side to side. Focus on reaching 70 percent of your maximum heart rate.

How-To: Make sure you have enough room to move side to side. Stand with your feet together, then take three steps to your right, and tap your left foot in, as pictured. Then take three steps to your left and tap your right foot in. Once you feel comfortable with the movement and spacing, pick up the pace. If it helps you to focus, you can put two objects on the floor to help measure your distance.

How Long: 1 minute, 3 times, with 10 seconds in between, for a total of about 3½ minutes

The Details:
- ▶ DO: Get your body low. Imagine that someone is going to toss you an egg at any moment. Don't let it drop and break.
- ▶ DO: Land softly with each shuffle.
- ▶ DO: Focus on your posture. Keep your hips and knees in alignment, as you move side to side.

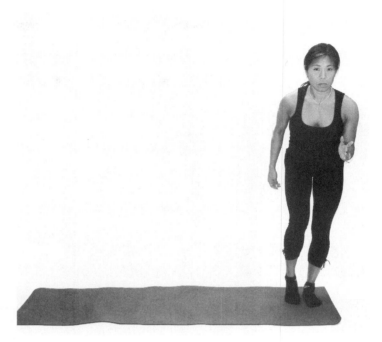

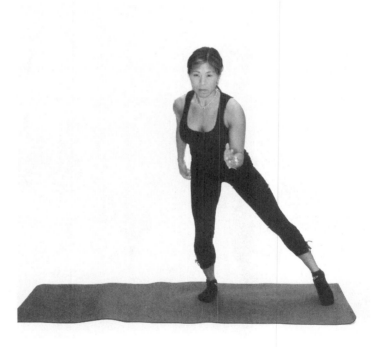

(continued on next page)

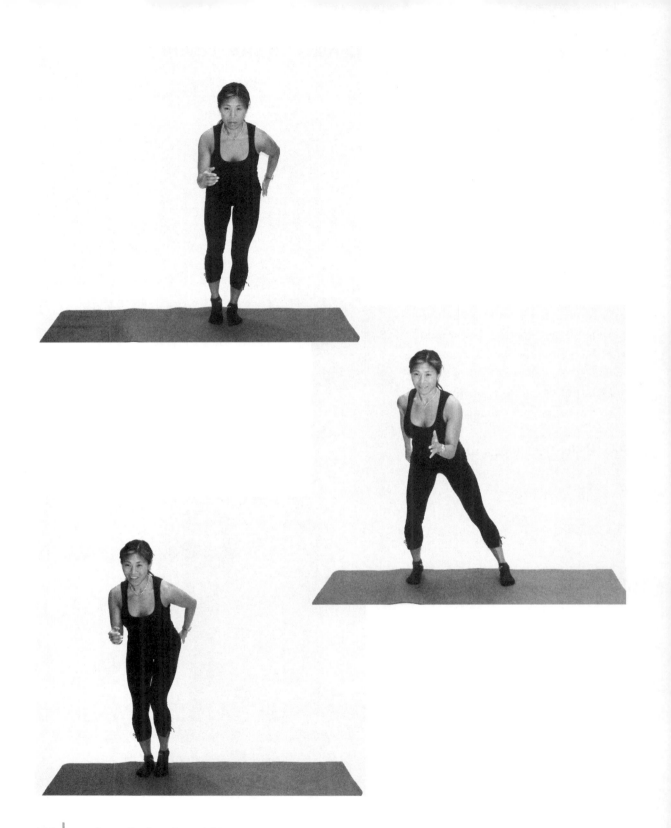

6. LUNGE-BALANCE WITH BICEP CURLS AND SHOULDER PRESS

Target: Butt, abs, biceps, and shoulders. Focus on each muscle with each movement.

How-To: Hold a dumbbell in each hand (men: 8–15 pounds; women: 3–10 pounds). Stand with your feet together, your arms by your sides, and your palms facing inward. Step back with one leg, as you lunge straight down, as pictured. Then come forward out of the lunge, back into the starting position. As you do this, perform a bicep curl, with your palms facing your shoulders, as pictured. Then press the dumbbells overhead, as you twist your palms, so that they face out. Slowly return your arms back to your sides. Then repeat with the other leg.

How Many: 10–15 with each leg, alternating

The Details:

▶ DO: Keep your weight in your front hip and heel. This makes you use your butt muscles as you lunge.
▶ DO: Move slowly, and with control, as you focus on each muscle group: those in your butt, your biceps, your abs, and your shoulders.
▶ DON'T: Arch your back as you press the weights overhead.
▶ DON'T: Put too much weight on the leg that steps back. It's only there to help with balance.

(continued on next page)

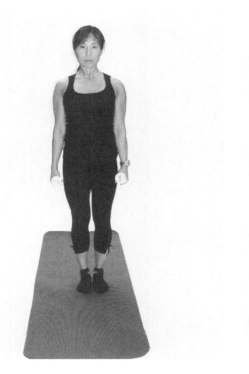
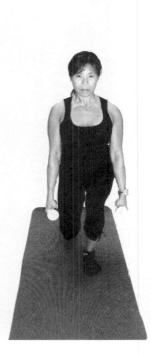

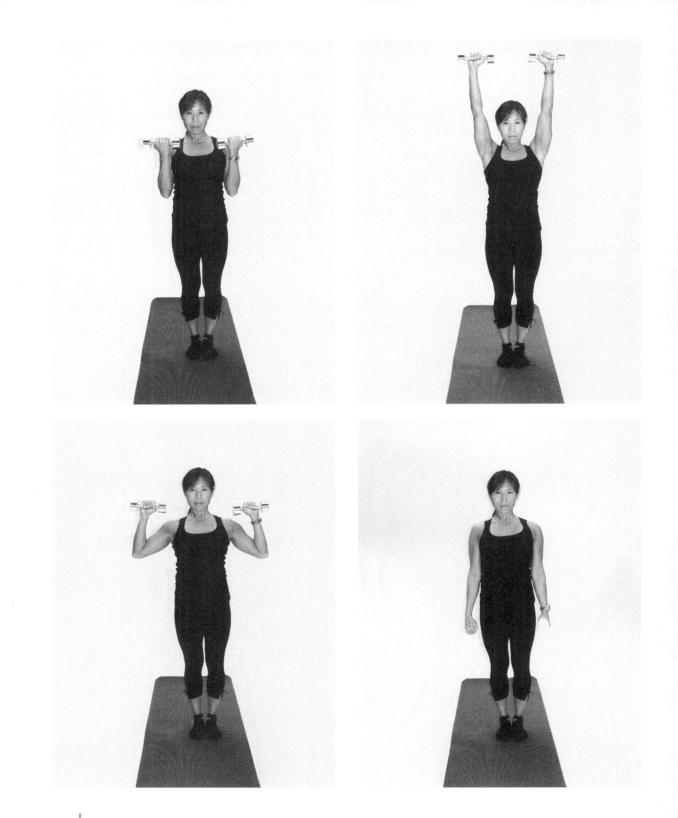

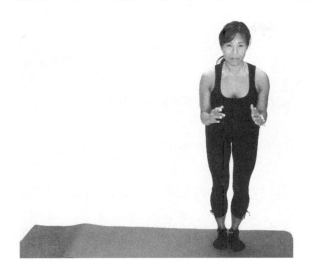

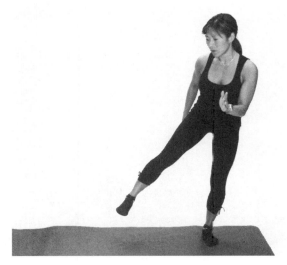

Target: Your butt, core, cardiovascular system, and ability to balance.

How-To: Stand with your feet together. Then step or jump laterally and land with your outside hip in a semisquat position, as pictured. Step the trailing foot in for balance, then step or jump in the other direction.

How Many: Do 20–30 jumps on each side—or 40–60 total. Do this 3 times.

The Details:

▶ DO: Keep your knee in a straight line above your big toe, to keep the work in your butt, instead of your knee.

▶ DO: Get your heel down as you land. Think of the movement as a one-legged squat.

▶ DO: Keep your head and chest up. Always keep good posture.

▶ DO: Use your arms to help you move and balance.

▶ DON'T: Lean forward, or stay on the balls of your feet.

▶ DON'T: Let your weight shift too much to each side. Keep your hips and knees in alignment.

▶ DON'T: Try to jump too fast. Always stay in control.

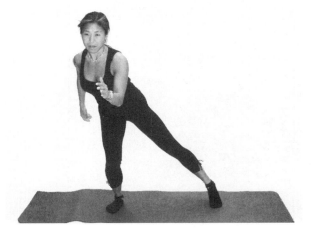

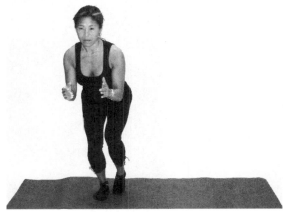

8. ABDOMINAL BICYCLE CRUNCHES

Target: Your abs.

How-To: Lie on the floor with your hands behind your head. Then raise your knees up to 90 degrees, as pictured. Curl your shoulders slightly off the floor to contract your abs. Look up at your knees and start to move your legs in a backward circular motion, as if you were riding a bicycle backward.

How Many: 40 complete pedals

The Details:

▶ DO: Hold your crunch position as you bicycle.
▶ DO: Try to keep your legs as close together as possible.
▶ DON'T: Use momentum. Focus on driving your torso into the ground with each movement.
▶ DON'T: Kick your legs straight out. Focus on creating a backward, circular motion. This engages your abs, not your hip flexors.
▶ DON'T: Pull on your neck or head as you hold the crunch position.

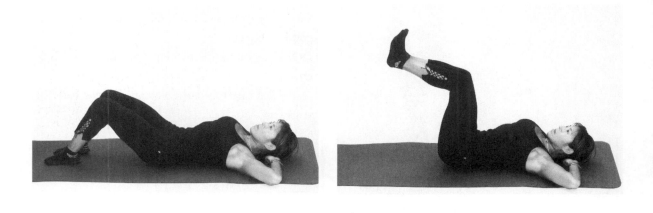

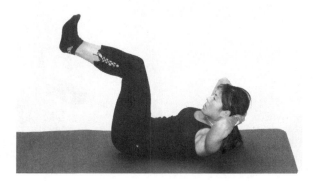

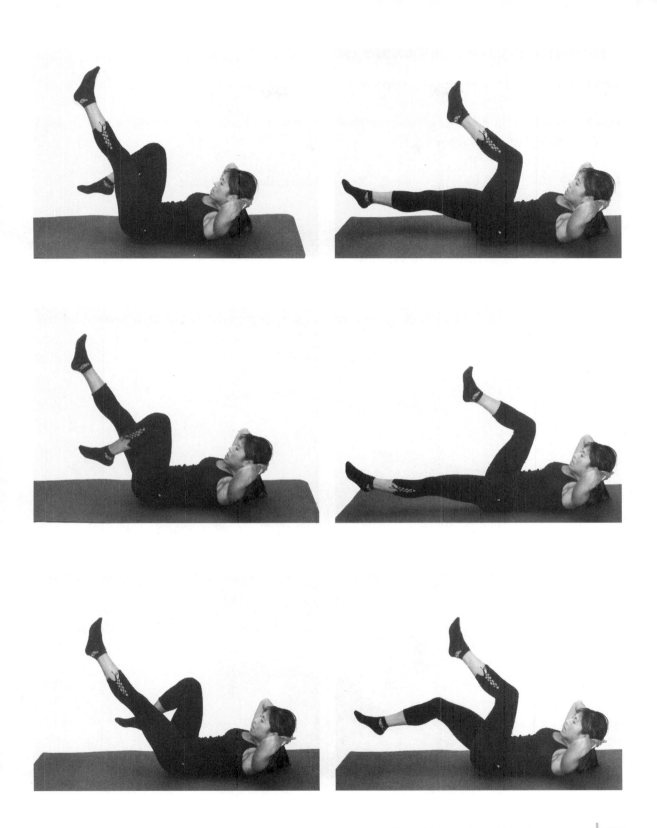

9. MOUNTAIN-CLIMBER CARDIO INTERVAL

Target: Your heart rate, and your abs, upper body, and core muscles.

How-To: In a push-up position, or on your elbows, as pictured, bend one knee in toward your chest. Then switch, and bring the other knee in.

How Many: 20 reps with each leg—40 total. Rest a moment, then do 40 more.

The Details:

▶ DO: Focus on your supporting leg—not on the knee that is coming in toward your chest.

▶ DO: Keep your back as flat as possible.

▶ DON'T: Shift your weight forward or backward with each climb. Try to remain steady, as if a glass of water were balancing on your back.

▶ DON'T: Let your shoulders collapse. Imagine you're trying to push the ground away from you as you support yourself.

In push-up position

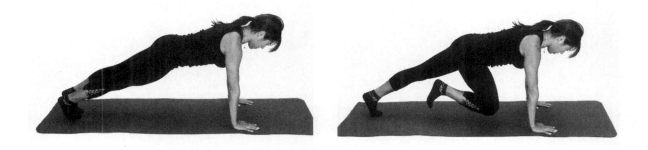

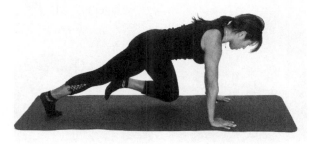

In elbows position

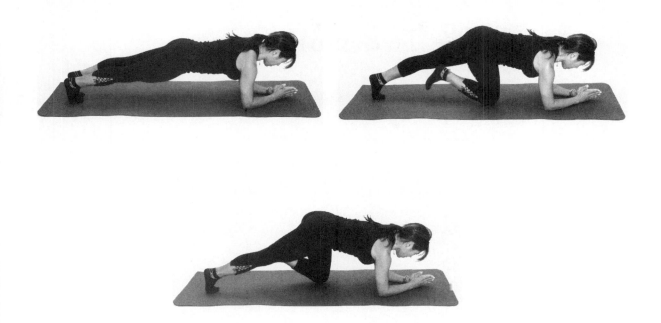

COOLDOWN

Do the usual. Just keep moving. Give yourself a pat on the back. The week is over. Carry your achievement into the weekend.

During the weekend, you get a break from your workouts. Enjoy it—but use it. Have fun with the new body that you're creating. Go for a long walk. Go swimming, biking, hiking, bowling. Play!

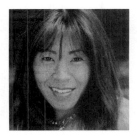

Yumi Lee, who helped design your core interval workout, is an internationally known aerobics competitor, and one of the top personal trainers in the entertainment industry. A Reebok University Master Trainer, Yumi was recently named one of "The 100 Best Trainers in America" by *Men's Journal* (along with Tanja Djelevic, and Greg). Her core training, kickboxing, and abdominal fitness classes at Crunch Fitness and Equinox Fitness are among the most popular fitness courses in Los Angeles. She has helped train Demi Moore, Sporty Spice, Brad Pitt, Peter Krause, and Pink, and she is a frequent contributor to *Glamour, Shape, Fitness,* and *Self.* Her very special workouts are known for challenging clients both mentally and physically.

Appendix **B**

The Phase Two Workouts

Welcome to the Phase Two Workouts

In Phase Two, you'll probably make your forays into the Breakthrough Moment—that difficult area in which further exercise feels impossible (but isn't). When you hit the Breakthrough Moment, your muscles will burn and quiver, and you'll want to stop. Try pushing beyond it.

I hope I'm not scaring you. Most of these exercises won't carry you to the Breakthrough Moment. They'll challenge you, but they're designed to be doable.

Remember: Don't quit before your half-hour is over: Obey the power of the Magic Half-Hour. If you finish all the exercises before a half-hour is over, repeat some of them, or do a vigorous post-workout cooldown. If you hit the half-hour mark before you finish the workout, it's okay to stop. But do try to get as many of the exercises done as possible, to involve all of your muscle groups.

Phase Two | **Monday** | *Strength Training Day*

WARM-UP

Do your standard 15-minute warm-up. Try to increase your heart rate by 50 percent; 70 percent is even better for this phase. Work up a sweat. Loosen up your muscles. Open your lungs.

Your 30-Minute Workout

1. SUPERMAN: Same exercise as in Phase One. Now, increase your duration. Do three 45-second holds, for a total of 2¼ minutes. Break them up, if necessary, into shorter increments.

2. SIDE BRIDGES: Same exercise as in Phase One. Now, increase your duration. Do 45 seconds on each side.

3. PULLOVERS: Same exercise as in Phase One. Now, do them with dumbbells. Men: Use 5 pounds in each hand. Women: 3 pounds. Focus on doing them more slowly. Increase your reps to 20.

4. TOTAL PUSH-UPS: Same exercise as in Phase One. Now, increase your reps to 10–15. Do them in smaller segments, if necessary.

5. OUTSIDE BICEP CURL: Same exercise as in Phase One. Now, increase your reps to 3 sets of 30. If you're a man, you should also increase the weight so that 30 reps are very challenging.

6. ACCORDION CRUNCH: Same exercise as in Phase One. Now, increase your reps to 3 sets of 20.

For Women Only: Greg's Lower-Body Blast

In Phase Two, you do a five-part set of exercises instead of three.

7A. PELVIC THRUSTS: Same exercise as in Phase One. Now, do 30 total reps, and hold every tenth rep for 10 seconds.

7B. SWEEP KICKS: Same exercise as in Phase One. Now, increase your output to 30 reps with each leg, and hold the thirtieth rep for 10 seconds.

7C. WALL SQUATS: Same exercise as in Phase One. Now, double your duration to a total hold of 90 seconds. Do it in increments, if necessary.

Target: Butt, thighs, and hamstrings.

How-To: With your feet shoulder-width apart and your knees slightly bent, bend over and stretch forward, as if you were diving into a swimming pool. Focus on your hamstrings—the thick muscles in the back of your thighs—and stretch forward until you can feel tension in them. Then, make a fist, squeeze your butt, and come back up.

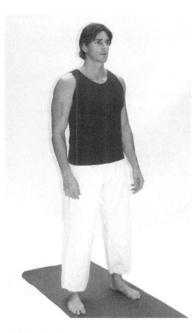

How Many: 15 reps

The Details:

▸ DO: Keep your back straight and knees slightly bent at all times to keep the power in your legs and butt.

▸ DO: Feel for tension in your butt, and keep it there, instead of in your back. Keeping your chin up will help you do this.

▸ DO: Spread your fingers as you move into the exercise, while you visualize the fibers of your hamstring muscles spreading and separating.

▸ DON'T: Rush the exercise. Doing so will strain your back.

▸ DON'T: Lock your knees.

▸ DON'T: Use your lower back—make your butt do the work.

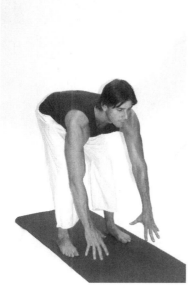

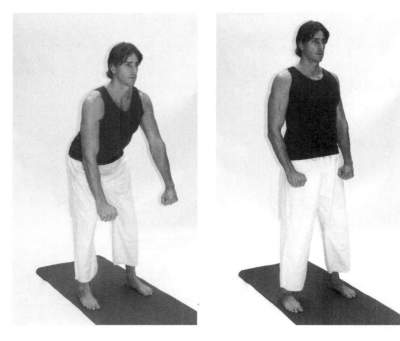

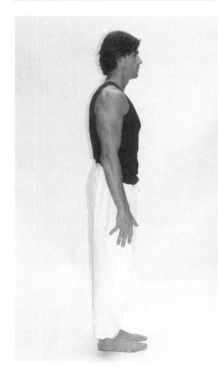

Target: Your butt.

How-To: Stand with your legs shoulder-width apart, then step slowly forward on one leg, as far as you can. As you step forward, slowly lower your other knee, but not all the way to the ground. Then come back up using your front heel and butt. Do it alternately with each leg.

How Many: 20 lunges

The Details:

▶ DO: Rise back up off your front heel, not your toes.
▶ DO: Lower with control, squeeze your butt as you lunge.
▶ DO: Focus mentally on gracefulness.
▶ DON'T: Clomp clumsily. Glide.
▶ DON'T: Let your front knee get ahead of your toes. Keep it behind them.

(continued on next page)

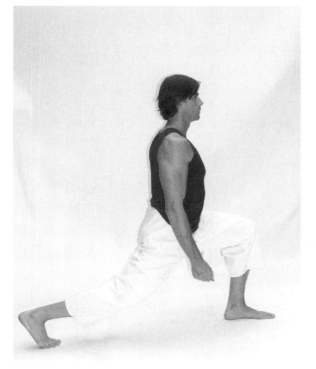

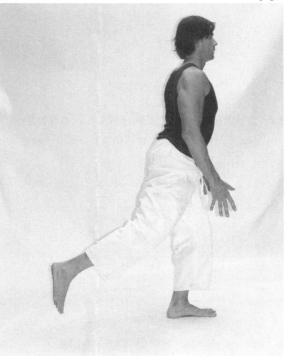

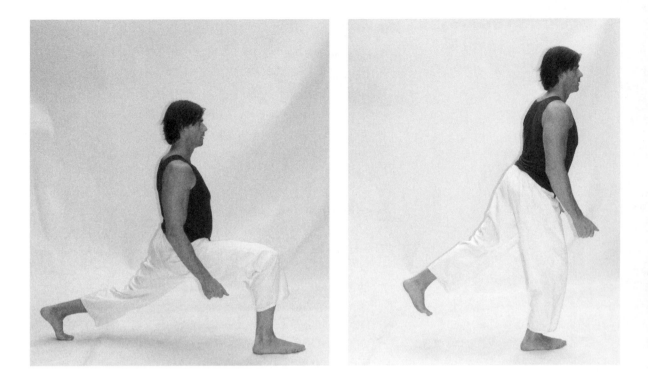

For Men Only: Greg's Upper-Body Blast

In Phase Two, you do a four-part set of exercises instead of three.

8A. SUPER TRICEP SKULL-CRUSHERS: Same exercise as in Phase One. Now, increase
   your reps to 20, with 10–15-pound weights.

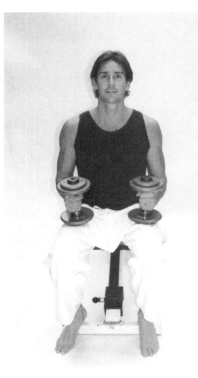

Target: Shoulders.

How-To: Sit on the edge of a bed or bench, with your dumb-bells shoulder-width apart. Push the weights straight up, and touch them together at the top. Lower them to your shoulders, and repeat.

How Many: 15 reps with 10–15 pounds

The Details:

▶ DO: Keep your chin straight to keep tension out of your back and neck.
▶ DO: Create a mental image of lifting the weights with your rib cage, in order to keep the work in your shoulders.
▶ DO: Squeeze your abs as you lift to protect your back.
▶ DON'T: Dig your chin into your chest.
▶ DON'T: Let your back bend or sway.

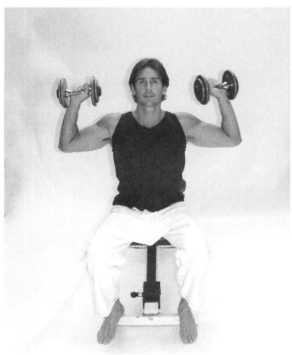

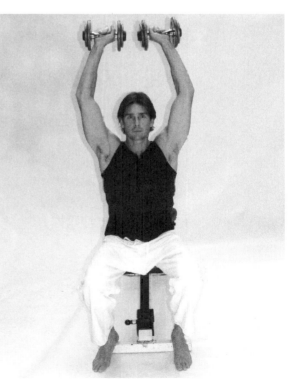

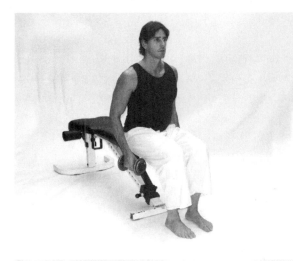

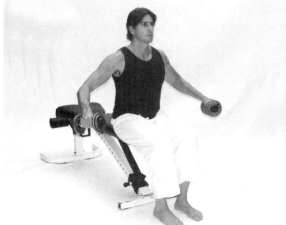

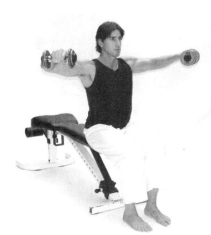

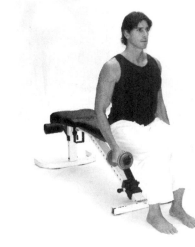

Target: Your shoulders—particularly your front and rear deltoids, and your shoulder cap.

How-To: As you sit, bend slightly forward, and raise both dumbbells, with your arms straight, as pictured.

How Many: 15 reps, with at least 5–10 pounds

The Details:

- ▶ DO: Focus mentally on pulling the dumbbells away from your body as you lift them.
- ▶ DO: Raise them on a count of 2, and lower them on a count of 5.
- ▶ DON'T: Arch your back.
- ▶ DON'T: Squeeze your neck.

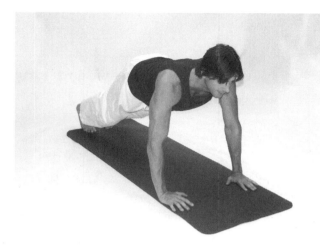

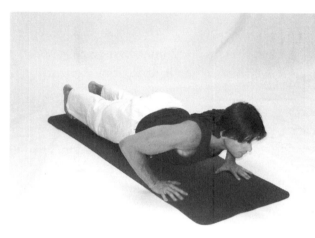

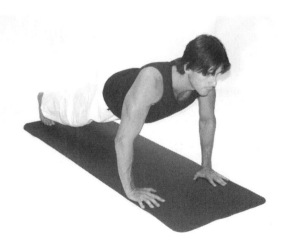

Target: Chest, shoulders, and triceps.

How-To: With your arms shoulder-width apart, your fingers spread, and your back straight, lower down on a 5-count, and then come back up on a 2-count.

How Many: Do as many as you can—this is called "repping out." Welcome to the Breakthrough Moment.

The Details:

▶ DO: Keep your proper form and pace. If you're not doing it right, you're not doing it.
▶ DO: Spread your fingers to help facilitate the flexion of your chest. This will work your chest more.
▶ DO: Squeeze your pecs throughout the exercise.
▶ DON'T: Let your back sag or arch. Keep the tension where it belongs—in your chest and arms.
▶ DON'T: Let your chin drop. Keep looking straight ahead.

COOLDOWN

Do the usual. Enjoy your accomplishment. Catch your breath. Stretch out. Unwind. Be in your body.

Phase Two | **Tuesday** | *Yoga Day*

WARM-UP

Push up your heart rate and warm up your muscles for about 15 minutes. Find something you really enjoy—like walking or riding your bike—and focus on the pleasure of it.

Your 30-Minute Workout

1. FORWARD BEND: Same movement as in Phase One. Now, increase your duration. Hold it for 3 minutes, in segments if necessary.

2. BOUND ANGLE POSE: Same posture as in Phase One. Now, try to go a little deeper, and push your duration from 2 minutes to 3 minutes.

3. HALF-PIGEON POSE: Same pose as in Phase One. Now, go for 2 minutes on each side, for a total of 4 minutes. If you hit the wall of the Breakthrough Moment too hard, do it in segments.

4. CAT COW BACK: Same posture as in Phase One. Now, increase your number of reps to 10.

5. DOWNWARD DOG POSE: Same pose as in Phase One. Now, increase your duration. Hold it for 3 minutes.

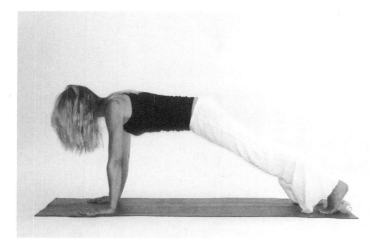

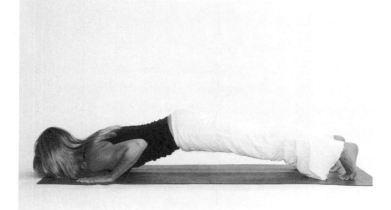

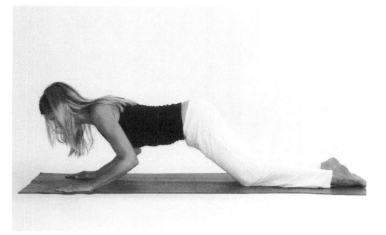

Target: Your arms—especially your shoulders and triceps.

How-To: From Downward Dog, move into a push-up position, as pictured. Inhale, and then exhale as you lower your body toward the floor. Tighten your abdominal muscles, and hold the position for 30 seconds. Try to hold your body off the floor with your elbows tucked in to your sides. Then push yourself up, and hold it at the top for another 30 seconds.

How Long: 30 seconds at the bottom of the pose.

The Details:

▶ DO: Keep your shoulders directly above your hands.
▶ DO: Lead with your chest and head as you lower your body toward the floor.
▶ DO: Put your knees on the floor if you have difficulty with the push-up, as pictured.
▶ DON'T: Sag. Keep your body almost straight, with your butt only slightly elevated. If you sag, you can hurt your back.
▶ DON'T: Lift your head—keep looking in front of you. If you lift your head, you can hurt your neck.

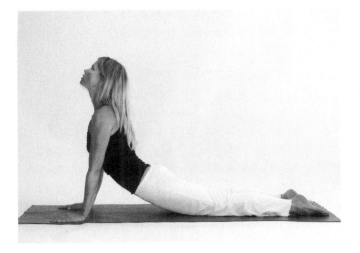

In knee position

Target: Your chest. The front of your shoulders. The muscles that support your spine.

How-To: Stay at the bottom of the push-up position, but put the tops of your feet flat onto the floor, as pictured. Lift your body up, as pictured, using your belly muscles for lift, and push your chest forward, with your head up. Hold that position.

How Long: Hold it for 30 seconds, 1 time.

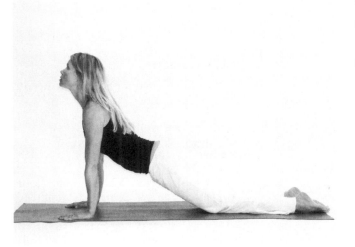

The Details:

▶ DO: Put your knees on the floor, if the posture is too difficult, as pictured.
▶ DO: Keep your arms extended, but without locking your elbows.
▶ DO: Stretch your spine, creating space between your vertebrae, before you arch up.
▶ DON'T: Let your back sag. It will strain it.
▶ DON'T: Hunch your shoulders up around your ears. That can strain your neck and shoulders.
▶ DON'T: Hyperextend. That can compress your vertebrae.

8. CHILD'S POSE: Same pose as in Phase One. This time, hold it for 3 minutes instead of 2.

9. SPINE TWIST: Same movement as in Phase One. Now, hold it for 1½ minutes on each side.

10. BRIDGE: Same posture as in Phase One. Now, hold it for 2 minutes, 2 times.

11. CORPSE POSE: Same posture as in Phase One. Stick with 5 minutes' duration.

COOLDOWN

After the Corpse Pose, which is your cooldown, move around a little and enjoy the new suppleness of your body.

Phase Two | Wednesday | *Pilates Day*

WARM-UP

Do a slightly shorter warm-up, because this Pilates workout will take longer than the workout in Phase One.

In Phase One, you did primarily supine moves, lying on your back with your face up. You'll do those again. In addition, in Phase Two, you'll add prone exercises, lying on your stomach with your face down. You'll also add standing position exercises. You've got a lot to get done—so let's hit it!

Your 30-Minute Workout

1. **SUPINE EXERCISES:** These are the same moves you did in Phase One, but now do the same number of reps—10 of each—in a flowing pattern, without resting in between them. If that's too difficult, do as many as possible without resting in between. Also, they should be done somewhat more quickly.

    Here is a review of the supine exercises from Phase One. If you don't remember exactly how to do them, see Phase One for the details.

    1. **Standing Roll-Downs (Note: These and Plié Squats are standing poses, but belong at the beginning of your workout.)**
    2. **Plié Squats**
    3. **Roll-Ups**
    4. **The Hundreds**
    5. **Single-Leg Stretches**
    6. **Straight-Leg Stretches**
    7. **Double Straight-Leg Stretches**
    8. **Rolling Like a Ball**

2. **PRONE EXERCISES:** When you have mastered these, they are supposed to be executed in a flowing manner, with less rest between sets. Managing to do these in a flow is an indicator of how much stronger you are becoming. Feel the flow, and feed it into the rest of the Workouts, and also your life.

Target: Your whole body.

How-To: Raise yourself into the Plank Position, as pictured, supporting yourself on your elbows and toes. Tuck your tailbone under, and pull your belly in toward your spine. Hold it.

How Long: Hold it for 30 seconds. Then rest on the floor for 30 seconds, and repeat the exercise, for a total of 5 lifts.

The Details:
▶ DO: Create a "turtle back" with your spine, by tucking your tailbone under.
▶ DO: Keep breathing. Breathe in on the exertion, and out on the release.
▶ DO: Take a break if your back starts to hurt.
▶ DON'T: Let your back sway.
▶ DON'T: Stick your butt in the air.
▶ DON'T: Let your chest or shoulders sag.

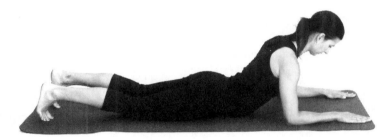

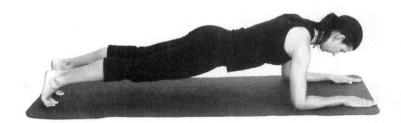

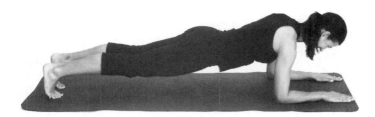

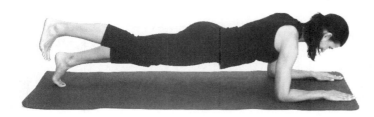

Target: Your butt. Your powerhouse.

How-To: Stay in Plank Position, and raise your right leg about 2 inches off the floor. Then put it back down, and raise the other leg.

How Many: Raise each leg 10 times.

The Details:

▶ DO: Keep flowing. Make it smooth and coordinated.

▶ DO: Keep your belly tucked in.

▶ DO: Stabilize your hips as you lift.

▶ DON'T: Sway your back. Keep the work in your powerhouse.

▶ DON'T: Drop your chin.

▶ DON'T: Lift your legs too high. That can hurt your lower back.

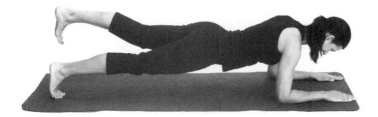

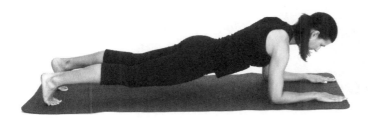

Target: Your whole body.

How-To: In the Plank Position, create a turtle back, as pictured, by tucking your tailbone in toward your abdomen. This is almost like doing an ab crunch, but in a prone position.

How Many: 10 reps

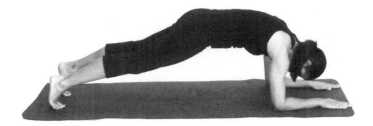

The Details:

► DO: Stay conscious of your abs and core.
► DO: Breathe in on the up movement and out on the down.
► DON'T: Sway your back, and drop your belly toward the floor.
► DON'T: Move your butt high up in the air.

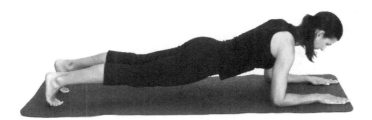

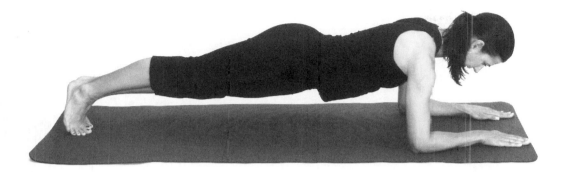

Target: Your entire body, with a focus on your lower back and your obliques.

How-To: In the Plank Position, move your feet close together, and twist your hips side to side, as pictured—almost as if you were dipping your hip down to the floor.

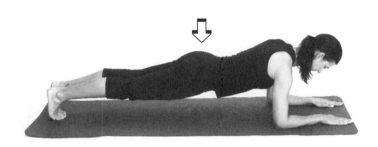

How Many: 10 twists on each side

The Details:

▶ DO: Keep your upper body completely stable. Don't shirk the work!

▶ DO: Tighten the muscles in your butt, and stay connected with your inner thighs. Mentally focus on the thought: *I'm lifting my body and my spirit.*

Now pause for a moment, in Child's Pose from Phase One's Yoga Day, which is much like the equivalent of the fetal position.

Next, go into the final portion of this workout: 5 Pilates standing-position exercises.

3. STANDING-POSITION EXERCISES

3A. KNEE PULL-INS

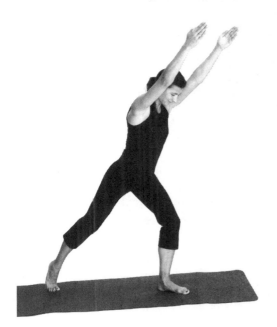

Target: Your powerhouse, along with your legs and arms. This movement also improves balance and grace.

How-To: Assume the pictured position. Then bring one knee in, as your arms move in toward your body. Then switch knees.

How Many: 10 reps with each knee

The Details:

▶ DO: Stay connected to every muscle. A lot of them are working here.

▶ DO: Make sure you initiate the exercise from your core's muscles.

▶ DON'T: Shrug your shoulders while you're moving your arms.

▶ DON'T: Slide your knees over your toes—it can eventually cause strain.

▶ DON'T: Rush. Take the time to do it right. If you're not doing it right, you're not doing it.

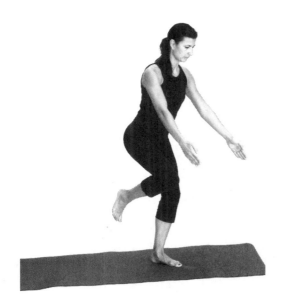

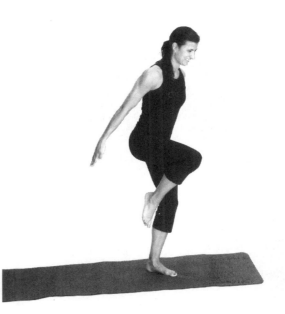

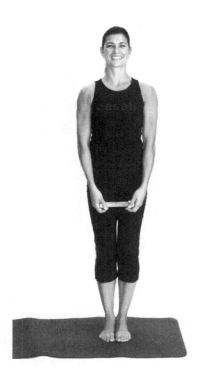

The Target: Your powerhouse, especially your butt. Also, your legs.

How-To: Stand in an upright position, holding a dumbbell with both hands, as pictured. Lunge with your leg to the side, while you reach for the floor with the weight. Then push away from the floor with your leg, shifting your weight back onto your heel. After that, reach overhead with the weight as you come back up to the starting position.

How Many: 10 reps with each leg

The Details:

- ▶ DO: Connect your mind to your whole body. This is an intense exercise!
- ▶ DO: Keep your back straight at all times. Protect it.
- ▶ DO: Keep your toes turned slightly out.
- ▶ DON'T: Be afraid to open your body, and expand it.
- ▶ DON'T: Say you can't. You can.
- ▶ DON'T: Shift your weight over your toes.

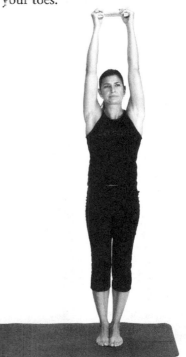

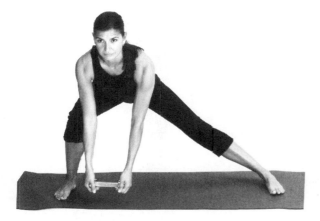

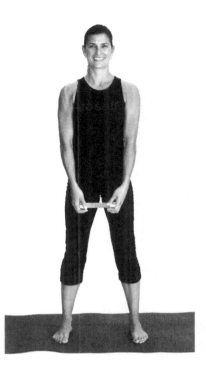

Target: Your whole body. Especially your powerhouse and legs.

How-To: Stand with your legs parallel and your feet hip-width apart, with a dumbbell between your hands, as pictured. Squat down, as if you were trying to sit in a chair, and put the weight down near the floor, without touching the floor. Then stand up, raise the weight overhead, and lift one knee, as pictured, to create a balancing pose.

How Many: 10 reps with each leg

The Details:

► DO: Shift back through your heels.
► DO: Keep your shoulders down.
► DO: Breathe from your powerhouse, and initiate the exercise from there.
► DON'T: Lean forward and arch your back.
► DON'T: Disconnect. Stay present. Stay focused.
► DON'T: Lock your knees.

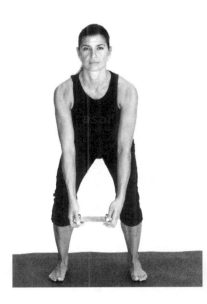

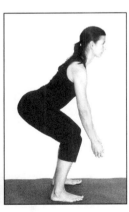

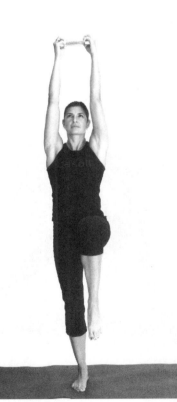

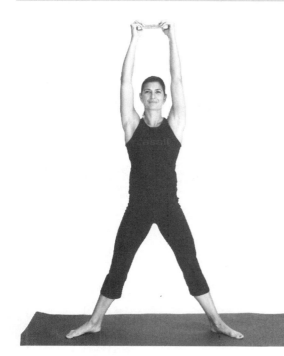

Target: Your whole body—as you'll soon see.

How-To: Do the same plié move you did in Phase One. This time, do it with a dumbbell between your hands, as pictured. While doing the plié, make a big circle with your arms holding the weight, as pictured, sweeping the floor and twisting your upper body.

How Many: 10 circles in each direction

The Details:

▶ DO: Inhale as you make a full circle, and exhale on a full circle.
▶ DO: Flow with your body. Feel it.
▶ DON'T: Keep your legs straight.
▶ DON'T: Arch your back.

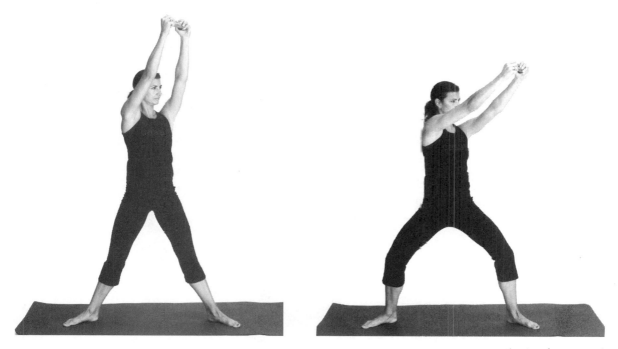

(continued on next page)

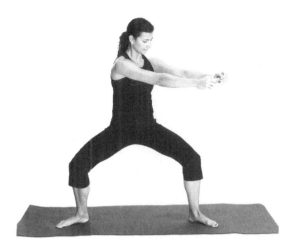

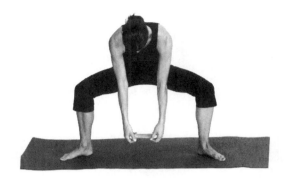

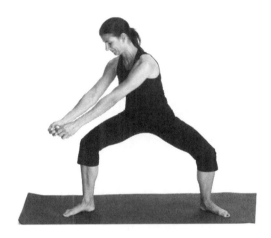

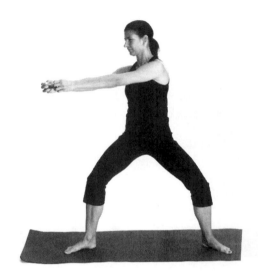

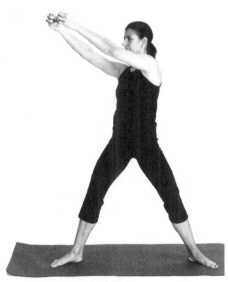

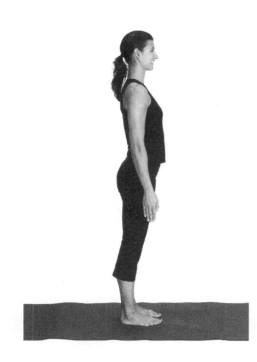

Target: Your whole body, and particularly your back and hamstrings.

How-To: Stand upright, in Neutral Position, and tilt forward with your arms reaching out, as pictured, and your leg reaching back—creating a T shape with your body. Hold it for 10 seconds. Come back to a standing position, with your arms down along your sides. Then do it with the other leg, holding that leg for 10 seconds also.

How Many: 10 reps with each leg, with 10-second holds

The Details:
- ▶ DO: Initiate the movement in your powerhouse.
- ▶ DO: Lower your shoulders and open your chest.
- ▶ DO: Find your ideal point of balance, and keep your limbs straight.
- ▶ DON'T: Hurry. Be mindful.
- ▶ DON'T: Tilt into more than the T position.

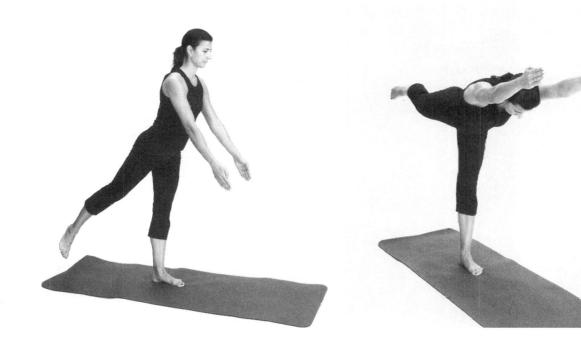

COOLDOWN

Keep moving for several more minutes. Go outdoors if the weather's nice. Stay connected to your body. Luxuriate in it!

Phase Two | **Thursday** | *Martial Arts Day*

WARM-UP

Do a slightly shorter warm-up, because the Phase Two workouts tend to take a little longer. But be sure to get loose. Martial arts can easily strain your muscles if they're tight. If you can't do all of this in 30 minutes, you may reduce the number of reps.

Your 30-Minute Workout

I. SHADOW BOXING

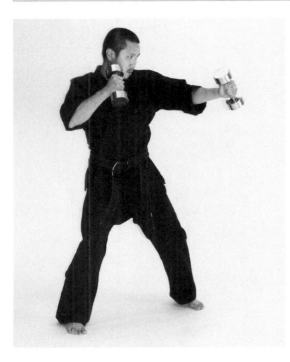

Target: Arms, shoulders, back, abs, and obliques.

How-To: Do it the same as in Phase One. But this time, do 20 reps of each of the 3 punches, instead of 15. This means:

▶ **Jab-Cross-Hook-Cross-Jab Combination.** This is a 5-punch combination that replaces the 3-punch combination you did in Phase One. It entails adding another cross and another jab at the end of the combination.

How Many: 20 Jabs. 20 Jab-Cross Combinations. Twenty of the 5-punch combinations with each hand leading, for a total of forty 5-punch combinations.

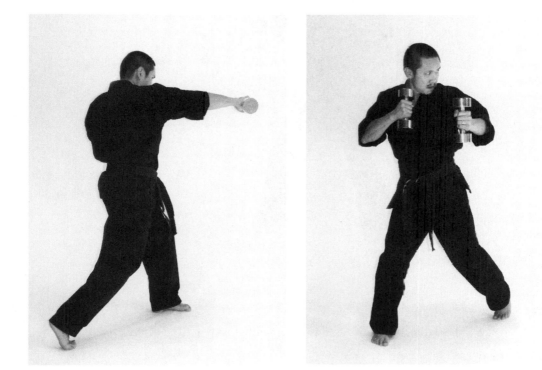

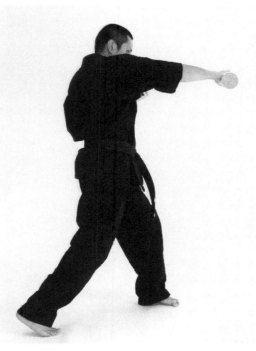

(continued on next page)

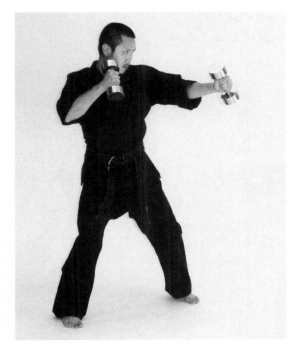

Remember: Do not hyperextend your arms. Always remember to practice accurate form.

Target: Your obliques and abs, and most of your leg muscles.

How-To: In Phase Two, you add a snap kick to the roundhouse kick to create a combination kick. First, do the snap kick. To do it, lift your knee, then quickly snap your foot forward, as if you were trying to strike an opponent in the groin. Then immediately do a roundhouse kick by bringing your knee to the V position, then quickly extending your leg, as pictured. Alternate the kicks—first snap, then the roundhouse—in smooth combinations. Do 20 reps of the combination with each leg. Then do 20 reps of just the roundhouse with each leg. Finish the last roundhouse kick by pulsing your leg upward 20 times.

How Many: 20 combinations with each leg. 20 roundhouse only, with each leg. 20 pulses.

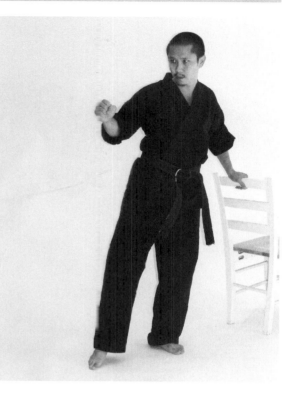

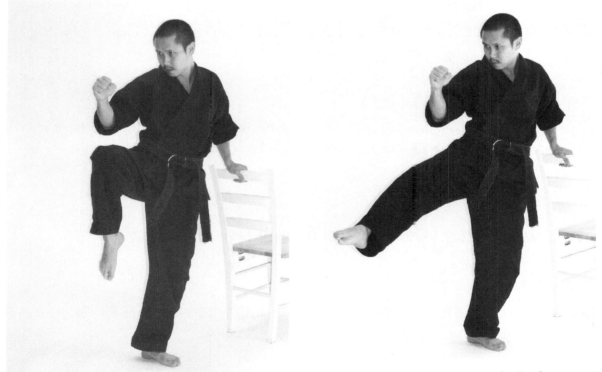

(continued on next page)

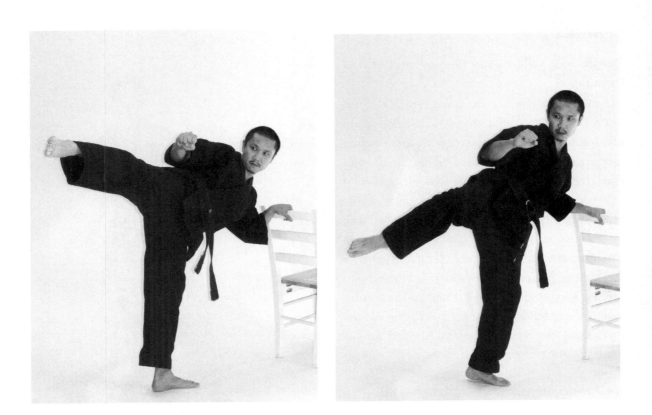

3. THAI KNEE-ABS

Same movement as in Phase One, but ratchet up your production to 3 sets of 15 reps, with each knee. Try to hit the Breakthrough Moment.

COOLDOWN

Don't be surprised if you're tired after this workout. Martial arts is fun, but really hits a lot of muscle groups. Stay active, stay loose, do some big breaths, and feel great.

Phase Two | **Friday** | *Core Interval Training Day*

WARM-UP

Do the same warm-up as in Phase One: 5 minutes of cardio, plus the 3-kick sequence. For a review of these kicks, see Phase One.

1. PUSH-UPS

Target: Your upper body and abs.

How-To: Same as in Phase One, but start with your legs hip-width apart. Also, this time, as you push up, extend one leg toward the ceiling, keeping your leg straight. Then bring that leg back down. Next, extend the other leg as you push up again.

How Long: 15 reps—or do it until you experience muscle fatigue.

The Details:

▶ DO: Focus on the supporting leg, to assist in the push-up.
▶ DO: Keep your abs engaged.
▶ DO: Keep your weight evenly balanced. Try not to shift all your weight to your supporting leg.
▶ DON'T: Overextend your leg, and arch your lower back.
▶ DON'T: Bend your knee as you extend your leg.

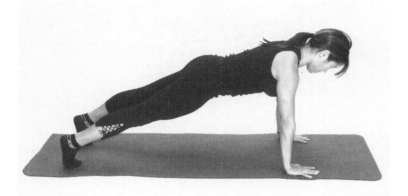

(continued on next page)

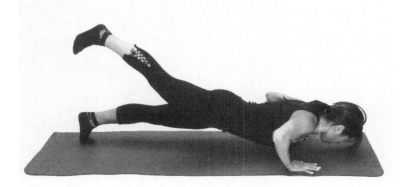

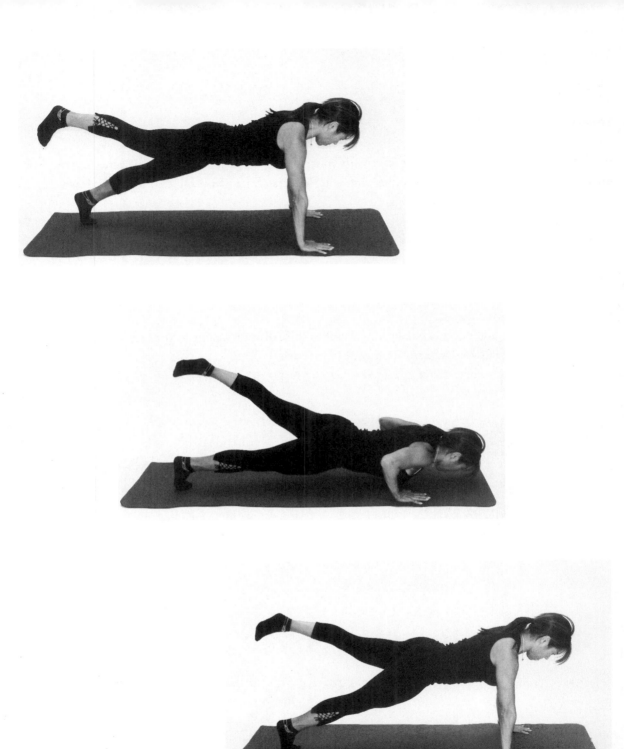

2. STATIONARY CARDIO INTERVAL

Target: Your heart rate. In this phase, push it up to about 75 percent of your maximum.

How-To: As in Phase One, do any movement—in place—that you can sustain at a moderate-to-fast pace: jumping jacks, jumping rope, or high knee lifts.

How Long: 1 minute, 3 times, with short breaks in between, for a total of 3 minutes

The Details:

▶ DO: Use your arms to increase the intensity. Push them overhead or in front, or to your sides.

▶ DO: Work harder than in Phase One. Don't cut yourself slack!

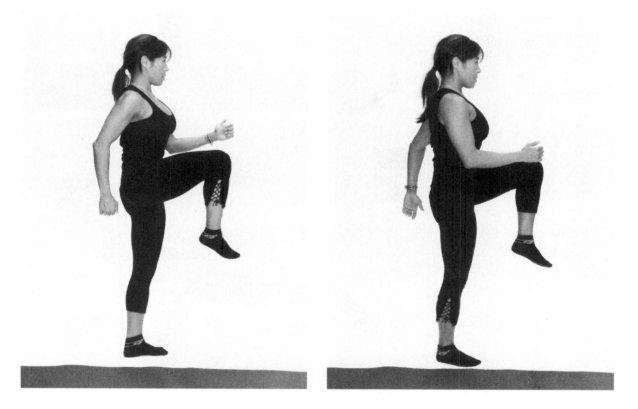

Target: Your upper back, shoulders, and abs.

How-To: Same as in Phase One—except now you will be standing only in a hinge position, on one leg, as pictured.

How Many: 8–10 with each leg

The Details:

▶ DO: Keep your supporting knee and hip bent.

▶ DO: Visualize driving your body's weight through the floor. This will help you maintain balance and stability as you reach and row.

▶ DO: Use a weight heavy enough to make your upper back and shoulder muscles work.

▶ DON'T: Use momentum. It will throw you off balance.

▶ DON'T: Arch your back. Try to keep your body flat and parallel to the floor.

▶ DON'T: Let your upper body lift out of the hinge as you row.

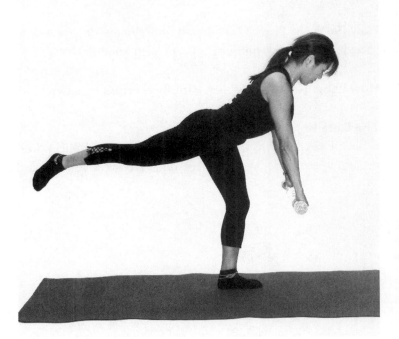

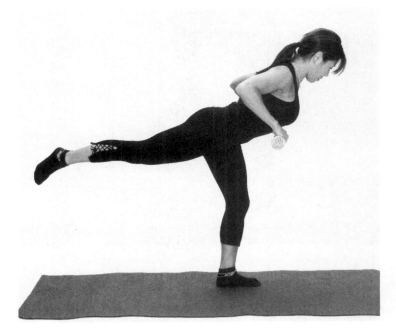

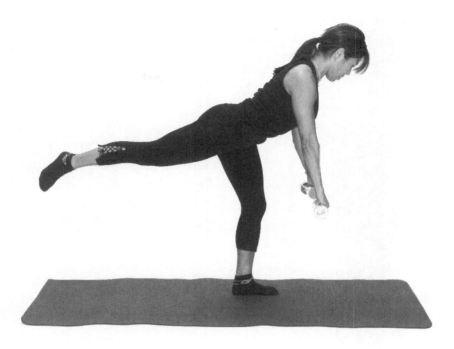

4. LATERAL-SHUFFLE CARDIO INTERVAL

Target: Your heart rate. Also, the muscles that control lateral movement. In this phase, try to hit 75 percent of your maximum heart rate.

How-To: Same as in Phase One. Now, though, focus on staying low, and on making quicker movements as you cover more floor space.

How Long: 1 minute, 3 times, with short rests in between, for a total of 3 minutes

The Details:
- ▶ DO: Really pick your feet up.
- ▶ DO: Keep your upper body steady and engaged.
- ▶ DON'T: Slide your feet across the floor.

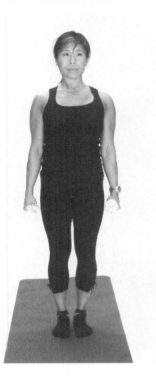

Target: Butt, abs, biceps, and shoulders. Focus on each muscle with each movement. Begin to incorporate more balance work.

How-To: Same as in Phase One. Now, though, as you step your feet together, put only your tiptoe down, as pictured, so that you are standing on your lunging leg when you perform the bicep curl. Then press the dumbbells overhead, as you twist your palms to face out. Slowly return your arms back to your sides, and repeat with the other leg.

How Many: 10–15 with each leg, alternating

The Details:

▶ DO: Keep your standing knee and hip slightly bent. This will give you more balance and stability.

▶ DO: Move slowly, and with control, as you focus on the specific muscle that you're working in your butt, your biceps, your abs, and your shoulders.

▶ DON'T: Arch your back as you press the weights overhead.

▶ DON'T: Push off your back leg as you stand up from the lunge. Drive through your supporting leg.

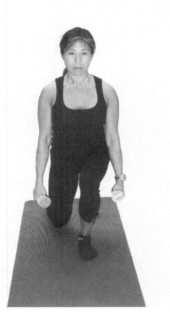

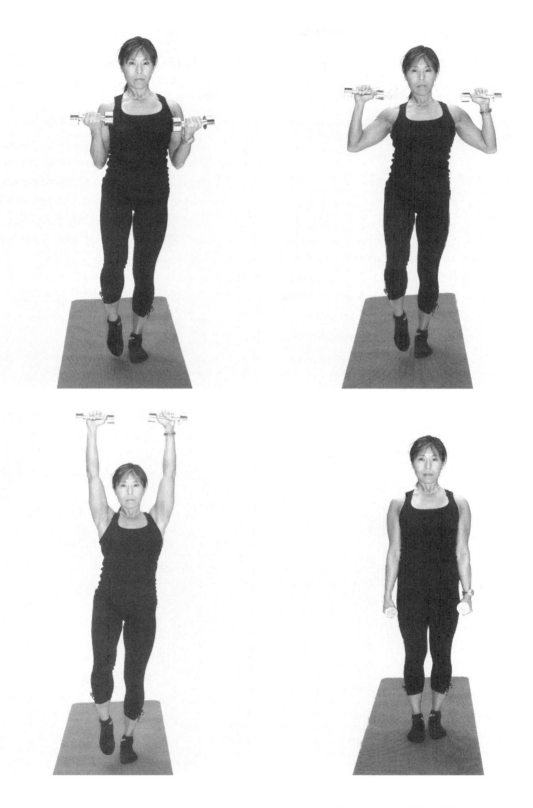

6. LATERAL-BOUNDING CARDIO INTERVAL

Target: Your heart rate—kick it up to about 75 percent of max. Also, your butt, core, and ability to balance.

How-To: Same as in Phase One. But now, as you land from the jump, barely tap the trailing toe, as you balance on one leg.

How Many: 20–30 jumps on each side—for 40–60 total. Do this 3 times. If you hit the Breakthrough Moment, try to push past it.

The Details:
- ▶ DO: Sink down into your supporting hip and heel as you land.
- ▶ DO: Keep your head and chest up. Visualize good posture.
- ▶ DO: Use your arms to help you move and balance.
- ▶ DON'T: Lean forward, or stay on the balls of your feet.
- ▶ DON'T: Try to jump too fast. Always stay in control.

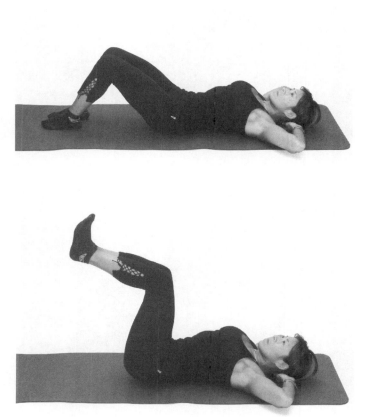

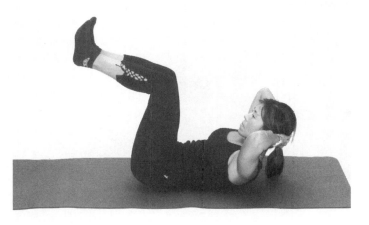

Target: Your abs and obliques.

How-To: Same as in Phase One, but add a twisting movement. As you bicycle your legs, rotate your upper body side to side, bringing your elbows to your opposite knees. Feel your abs stabilize, as your obliques work, while you twist.

How Many: 20 pedals with each leg, for a total of 40

The Details:

▶ DO: Keep your elbows open to the side as you rotate.
▶ DO: Try to keep your legs as close together as possible.
▶ DO: Try to keep your lower body centered, while your upper body rotates. It helps to visualize keeping your torso grounded, as you move slowly and with control.
▶ DON'T: Kick your legs straight out. Focus on creating a backward, circular motion, to use your abs, instead of your hip flexors.

(continued on next page)

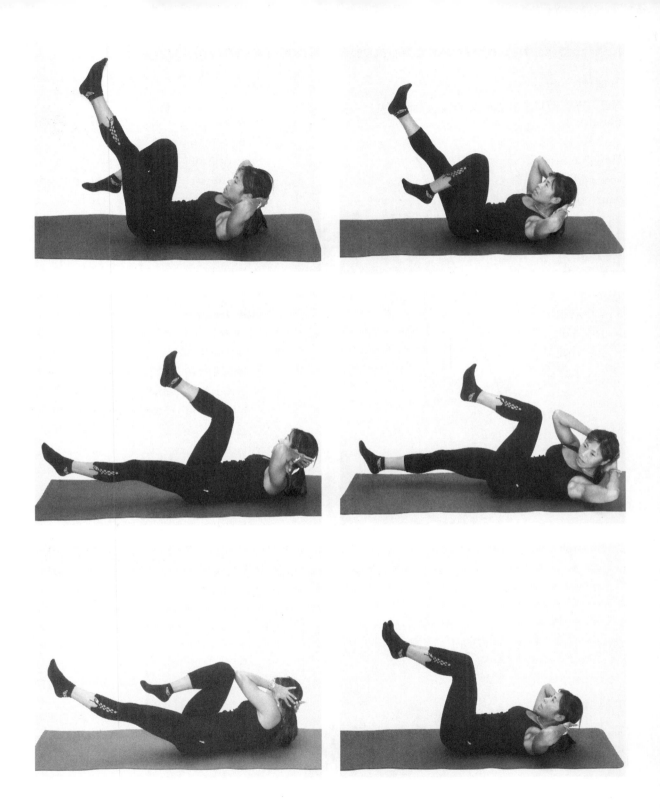

8. MOUNTAIN-CLIMBER CARDIO INTERVAL, WITH TWISTS

Target: Your heart rate: 75 percent of max. Also, your abs, upper body, and core muscles.

How-To: Same as in Phase One, but now you add twists. Bring your knee across your body toward the opposite elbow, as pictured.

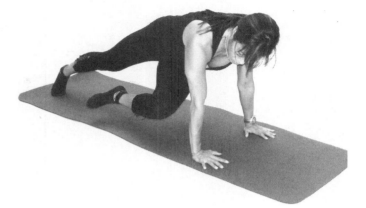

How Many: 20 reps with each leg, for a total of 40. Do it 2 times.

The Details:

▶ DO: Focus on the supporting leg, not the knee that is coming in toward the opposite elbow.

▶ DO: Keep your back as flat and stable as possible.

▶ DON'T: Let your hips drop as you twist.

▶ DON'T: Shift your weight forward or backward with each climb. Try to remain steady.

▶ DON'T: Let your shoulders collapse. Imagine you're trying to push the ground away from you, as you support yourself.

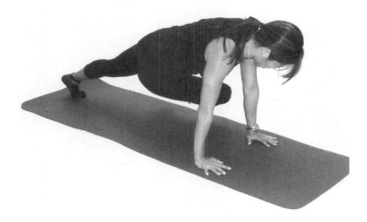

COOLDOWN

Take a short walk and reflect on your week. You've made real progress, haven't you? By now, you should be feeling stronger and leaner. Doesn't it feel great?

Another weekend is coming. Stay active. Have fun. The more you use your body, the better you will feel.

Since you're going to do a cleanse this weekend, don't worry about being too active. Focus on the cleanse.

The Phase Three Workouts

Welcome to Phase Three Workouts

You may spend more time in the Breakthrough Moment than you'd like in Phase Three, but every second you spend there really pays off. Besides, after a month of this, you're probably to the point where you would like a little Breakthrough Moment action every day. It gets your adrenaline going, and makes you feel like Superman when you're done.

Hang in there. This is a pivotal stage. The next two weeks could be one of the most important two-week periods of your life.

If you can get past the Phase Three workouts, you'll never be quite the same person.

As you did in Phases One and Two, keep exercising for a half-hour. If you can't get all the suggested exercises done in a half-hour, try doing fewer reps, or eliminate a few of the exercises. Better yet, at this stage, go over a half-hour.

You've already changed your body. Now change your life.

WARM-UP

Do the usual 15 minutes. Get warm and loose. Push your heart. Push your lungs.

Your 30-Minute Workout

I. SUPERMAN: Same exercise as before, but increase your duration again.
   How Long: 3 1-minute holds would be excellent. Any hold over 1 minute would be amazing.
   Perfect the details: Keep extending, up and out. Toes spread. Belly taut. Butt tight. No strain in your lower back or neck. Keep breathing. When it gets tough, wiggle your toes and fingers, or make a sound—like "ahhh"—from your belly.

2. SIDE BRIDGES: Same exercise as before, but increase your duration again.
   How Long: 1 full minute on each side. If you can do more than 1 minute, you've made great progress.
   Perfect the details: Keep your body rigid. Keep extending. Don't dig your shoulder in. Suck your belly in. Squeeze your butt.

3. PULLOVERS: Same exercise as before, but increase your output again.
   How Many: 25 reps, with dumbbells (men: 5 lbs, women: 3 lbs). If you've got the energy, go ahead and rep out. Break your own record. Live in the Breakthrough Moment.
   Perfect the details: If the weights get too heavy, put them down, but keep going. Draw in your stomach. Chin up. Be graceful. Keep a steady pace. Don't sacrifice good form.

4. TOTAL PUSH-UPS: Same exercise as before, but increase your reps again.
   How Many: 15 to 20 reps. If you can break 20, keep going until your arms burn. Well done.
   Perfect the details: Exaggerate the key elements of the exercise. Keep your stomach tucked in when you're at the top. Go low as early and as long as possible. When you go up, visualize reaching up and out with your chest.

5. OUTSIDE BICEP CURL: Same exercise as before, but increase it to your maximum possible number of reps.

6. ACCORDION CRUNCH: Same exercise as before, but increase your reps again.
   How Many: 3 sets of 25. Or really push yourself into the Breakthrough Moment, and go for 3 sets of 30–35.
   Perfect the details: Stretch your lower stomach without arching your back. Push your limits by stretching your belly an extra 2–3 inches. Keep breathing. Reach for the tops of your knees.

For Women Only: Greg's Lower-Body Blast

In Phase Three, you do a five-part Blast.

7A. PELVIC THRUSTS: Same exercise as before, but increase your reps again.

> **How Many:** 40 total reps, with a 10-second hold on every tenth rep, would be excellent. 50 or more would be amazing.

> **Perfect the details:** Tuck your glutes in—they're your power. Keep your back straight. Squeeze your butt. Don't arch your back. Feet flat, no matter what. Extension has to come from your butt, and nowhere else.

7B. SWEEP KICKS: Same exercise as before, but increase your reps again.

> **How Many:** 40 reps, with a 10-second hold on the thirtieth and fortieth reps, is excellent. 50 or more is really terrific!

> **Perfect the details:** Keep your toes pointed down, and lead with your heel. Make sure your hip is slightly rolled over, to help keep tension in your butt. Extend each kick above parallel. Don't bounce or flail. Go down slowly, and explode upward.

7C. WALL SQUATS: Same exercise as before, but increase the duration again.

> **How Long:** $2^{1}/_{2}$ minutes. If you can go 4 minutes, you're on your way to ultra-fitness.

> **Perfect the details:** Keep your arms above parallel and extended away from your body. Don't tense your neck. Chin up. When it gets tough, wiggle your extremities, or make a noise. Focus. Connect. Stay present.

7D. GOOD MORNINGS: Same exercise as before, but increase your reps again.

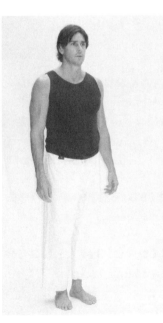

> **How Many:** 25 reps is great. 40 is beyond great. It's Breakthrough Moment great.

> **Perfect the details:** When you extend forward, pull your stomach in. Don't lock your knees—keep them bent. Come up from your butt, with the specific purpose of working your butt, instead of your lower back. Keep looking forward, not down. Go slow. This exercise is about connection, not speed.

7E. WALKING LUNGE

Same exercise as before, but now you add a snap kick to it. As you come out of your lunge, and bring your back leg up and forward, do a snap, karate-like kick before your next stride.

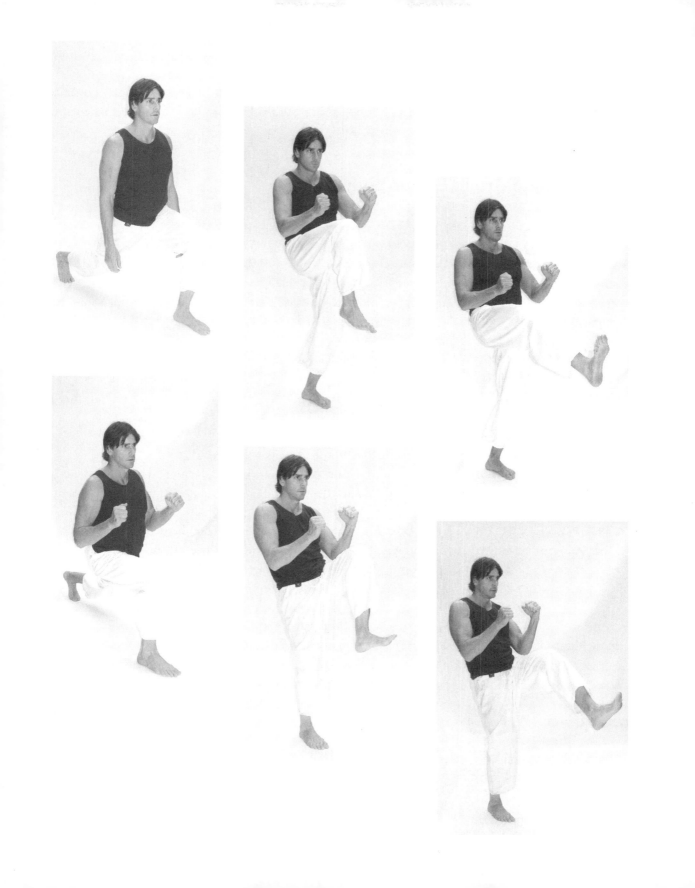

How Many: 20 lunges. If you can do 20 with a 5-pound dumbbell in each hand, you're doing fantastic.

Perfect the details: The key to the lunge is the length of the stride. Make it as long as possible. Don't drag your back foot—bring it through with purpose. Dig in your front heel when you kick. Snap with grace and connectedness.

For Men Only: Greg's Upper-Body Blast

In Phase Three, you do a five-part Blast. Please note the sequence has changed.

8A. OUTSIDE BICEP CURL: Same exercise as before, but increase your reps again.
   How Many: 25 reps with 10–15 pounds. Anything over that is fantastic.
   Perfect the details: Go as heavy as possible with your weights, without sacrificing form. Shoulders back. Chin up. Squeeze your pinkie instead of your thumb, into the dumbbell.

8B. MILITARY PRESS: Same exercise as before, but increase your reps again.
   How Many: 20–25 reps with 10–15 pounds.
   Perfect the details: Chin straight. Chest out. Straight back. Control your downward motion. Keep a steady pace.

8C. LATERAL FLYS: Same exercise as before, but increase your reps again.
   How Many: 15 reps with dumbbells, followed immediately by 15 more without weights.
   Perfect the details: Arms straight. Chin straight. Chest out. Bend forward with your back straight.

8D. SUPER TRICEP SKULL-CRUSHERS: Same exercise as before, but increase your reps again.
   How Many: 30 reps, with 10–15 pounds. If you really want to hit your triceps, shoot for 50.
   Perfect the details: Keep the tension in your muscles, not your joints. Squeeze your triceps. Don't check out and fall into lazy form. Your triceps should be on fire by the end of this.

8E. REP-OUT PUSH-UPS: Same exercise as before, but break your personal record from Phase Two.
   How Many: 30–40 is more than most people can do. More than 50 is a real achievement.
   Perfect the details: Straight back. Slow pace. Never sacrifice form for reps. It's not about reps—it's about the pace and connecting to your body.

COOLDOWN

Try to do some stretching in your Strength Training Day cooldown. Make those new muscles feel good. Welcome them like new friends.

WARM-UP

Push up your heart rate and warm up your muscles for only about 15 minutes. You'll need the extra time for the workout. Be more aggressive than you were in the first two phases. You've worked hard to get to this point, so make the most of it.

Your 30-Minute Workout

1. **FORWARD BEND:** Same posture as before, but increase your duration to 4 minutes—in increments, if necessary.

   Perfect the Details: Don't bend your knees—keep your legs straight. Push down with your inside thigh. Flex your little toe toward you.

2. **BOUND ANGLE POSE:** Same posture before, but increase your duration to 4 minutes—in increments, if necessary.

   Perfect the Details: Let your knees unfold, and open your hips. For variety, try lying down flat, and feeling the flavor of the pose in that position. If necessary, put a pillow under your knees, to make it a little easier.

3. HALF-PIGEON POSE

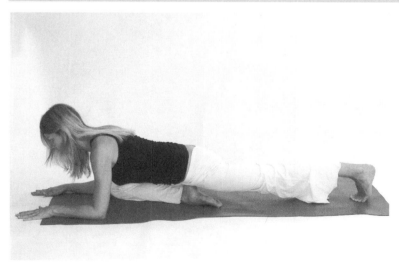

Same pose as before, maintaining your duration of 2 minutes on each side—in increments, if necessary.

Perfect the details: On the last minute of the posture, uncurl the toes of the leg that is behind you, and lift that knee off the ground. Then push back through your heel, to feel the opening of your hips. Then repeat it on the other side.

4. CAT COW BACK: Same posture as before, but now increase your reps to 15.

Perfect the Details: Focus on tucking your tailbone under, to create vertebral space. Also, visualize the lengthening of your lower back. But don't hyperextend.

5. DOWNWARD DOG POSE: Same pose as before, but now hold it for a full 5 minutes—in increments, if you can't bust past the Breakthrough Moment.

Perfect the Details: Visualize the inverted V shape. Keep your arms and legs strong. Squeeze your muscles throughout the posture. Lengthen your spine—really stretch it.

6. SUN SALUTATION

This is a combination of 5 poses. Go directly from one to the next.

Target: The entire body. This set of 5 postures brings heat and chi to your whole being, and facilitates your flow of energy.

How-To:

1. **Start with Mountain Pose,** as pictured, standing straight, with your heels and toes together, and your hands in Prayer Pose. Then inhale, squeeze your thigh muscles, feel a stretch in your spine as you reach your arms high over your head. Look up toward your hands.

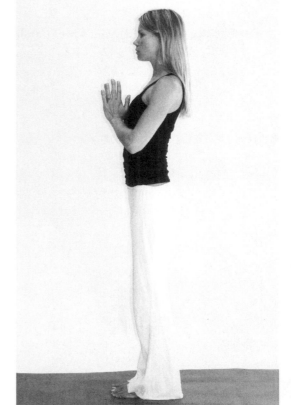

2. Then go into Forward Bend, exhaling as you hinge forward from your hips. Go all the way down, as pictured, until your hands can touch the floor, and your head is level with your knees. Then inhale, look up, lift your chest, and run your hands up behind your legs, to just below your knees. If your hamstrings are tight, bend your knees.

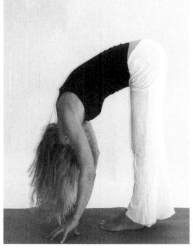

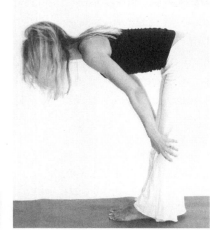

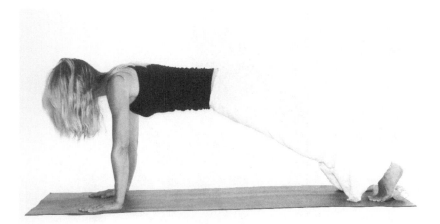

3. Exhale, and go into the top of the Plank Position. Lower your body toward the floor, keeping your abdomen engaged, and try to hold your body off the floor.

4. Inhale, then move into Upward Dog, lifting your torso off the ground, as pictured. Bring the tops of your feet flat onto the floor. Keep your head up, and your knees off the floor.

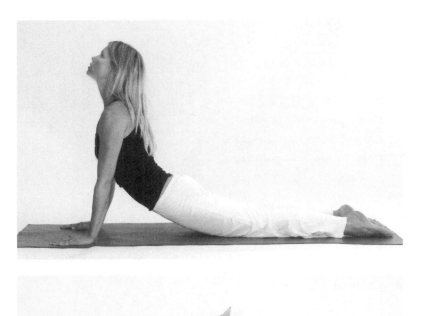

5. Finally, exhale to Downward Dog. Turn your toes back under, and go into the inverted V shape. Then pause and take five breaths here. Then inhale, step to the front of your mat into Mountain Pose. Start again.

How Long: Do this set of 5 postures 5 times. Each Sun Salutation should take about 1–1½ minutes.

The Details:
- ▶ DO: Keep your core muscles engaged at all times, to protect your lower back.
- ▶ DO: Practice your *ujjayi* breathing.
- ▶ DO: Rest in Child's Pose, if this becomes too difficult.
- ▶ DON'T: Hold your breath. Use your breath to move gracefully from one posture to the next, and to facilitate the flow of chi.
- ▶ DON'T: Hyperextend. Stretch without straining.
- ▶ DON'T: Close your eyes. Energy flow will be greater with your eyes open.

7. CHILD'S POSE: Same posture as before, but now hold it for 7 minutes.

Perfect the Details: Keep your elbows off the ground. Stretch your arms out. Push your tailbone back toward your heels, and really feel the stretch, all the way from your fingers to your tailbone.

8. CORPSE POSE: Same posture as before, but increase your duration to 10 minutes.

Perfect the Details: If you're feeling agitated, from cleansing or from another source of stress, do this with your legs propped up against a wall, to increase blood and energy flow to your head. To help bring energy to your chest and heart, put something like a pillow under your shoulder blades and head.

COOLDOWN

Your Corpse Pose is your cooldown. As you finish it, come into a comfortable cross-legged seat, taking your hands into Prayer Pose. Breath is life! Take a deep breath, and as you exhale, bow your head toward your heart, and say a prayer of thanks. *Namaste.*

Phase Three | **Wednesday** | *Pilates Day*

WARM-UP

Do whatever feels good. Just get your heart going, your muscles loose, and your lungs open. Don't wear yourself out, though. Energize yourself—you'll need it.

Your 30-Minute Workout

I. SUPINE EXERCISES: Do the 8 supine exercises you did in Phases One and Two, but now do them with 2-pound weights on your wrists or in your hands. And do them even a little faster than you did in Phase Two. Do 10 reps of each one.

PERFECT THE DETAILS

I. Standing Roll-Downs: Tuck your chin. Hold in your belly. Take your time.

2. Plié Squats: Stay straight—don't lean forward. Focus on grace. Connect to your breath.

3. Roll-Ups: Don't rush it. Live in your vertebrae.

4. The Hundreds: Stay rhythmical. Keep your chest up.

5. Single-Leg Stretches: Hips stable. Keep your pulse quick.

6. **Straight-Leg Stretches:** Feel each twist. Don't sway your back.

7. **Double Straight-Leg Stretches:** Stay under control. Don't lose touch with your abs.

8. **Rolling Like a ball:** Chin tucked, knees tight to your body. Don't let your feet touch the floor.

2. PRONE EXERCISES

2A. TRICEP PUSH-UP

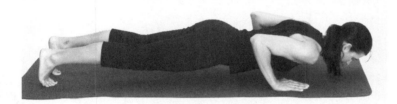

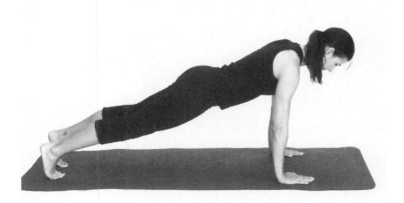

Target: Your powerhouse, your arms, your chest, and much of the rest of your body.

How-To: Get in a push-up position, as you did during Strength Training Day, but keep your arms close to your body. Move down toward the floor, keeping your elbows close to your sides. Come back up.

How Many: 15 reps. Do them in segments, if necessary. Aim for the Breakthrough Moment.

The Details:
- ▶ DO: Exhale as you go down, and inhale as you go up.
- ▶ DO: Engage your powerhouse.
- ▶ DON'T: Drop your belly all the way down to the floor.
- ▶ DON'T: Shrug your shoulders.
- ▶ DON'T: Point your elbows out from your body.

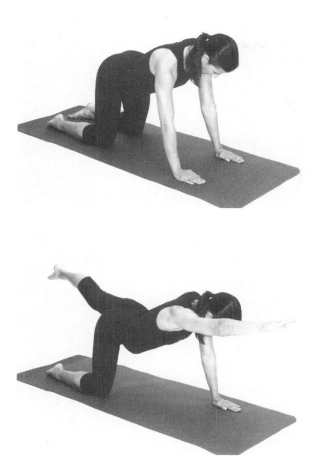

Target: Abs, back.

How-To: As in the yoga form of this exercise, get on your hands and knees, and reach your right arm out, with your left leg behind you, as pictured. Arch your back as your leg and arm meet under your body. Then extend your leg and arm again. Do it on each side.

How Many: 10 reps on each side

The Details:
- ▶ DO: Inhale on the pull-in and exhale on the push-out.
- ▶ DO: Keep your back straight.
- ▶ DO: Keep your powerhouse engaged.
- ▶ DON'T: Check out. Keep your mind and body together.

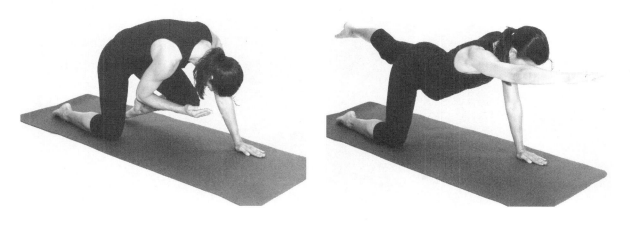

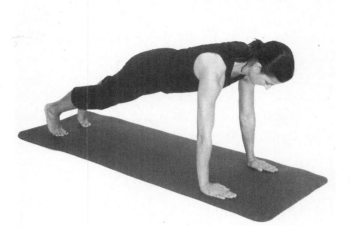

Target: Your whole body, concentrating on your lower abs and lower back.

How-To: Get in a push-up position, as pictured. Don't lift your butt. Then pull one knee in underneath you, bring it back out, and pull in the other knee.

How Many: 15 reps with each knee

The Details:
- ▶ DO: Keep your upper body stable.
- ▶ DO: Inhale on 2 counts, and exhale on 2 counts.
- ▶ DON'T: Disconnect. Stay with it. Be in your body.

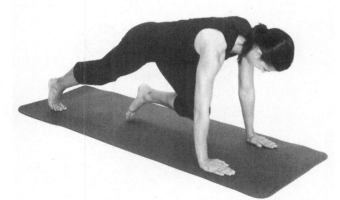

3. STANDING-POSITION EXERCISES

Do the same 5 exercises as in Phase Two, but try to do them more quickly, without sacrificing form.

PERFECT THE DETAILS

1. Knee Pull-Ins: Keep the work in your powerhouse. Don't shrug your shoulders.

2. Side Lunges: Connect your mind and body. Rise to the challenge.

3. Squat, Balance, Reach: Stay in your powerhouse—everything starts there. Shoulders down. Back straight.

4. Plié with Rotation: Go with the flow of the movement. Focus on grace.

5. Balance T Pose: Find the perfect point of balance. Don't hurry. Enjoy the effort.

COOLDOWN

Take it easy. You deserve it. You've taken care of your core today, so stretch your legs with a walk. Feel how much easier it is to walk briskly now than it was just a few weeks ago. You're getting there!

Phase Three | Thursday | *Martial Arts Day*

WARM-UP

Cut your warm-up down to 10 minutes. You'll need some extra time to do the workout. But make sure you do enough to get your muscles warm and loose.

Your 30-Minute Workout

1. PUNCH-AND-KICK COMBINATIONS: In Phase Three, you graduate to a series of 3 strenuous punch–kick combinations.

A. JAB-CROSS COMBINATIONS: This is the same combination you did in Phase One. Do it while holding weights, and increase your reps to 25.

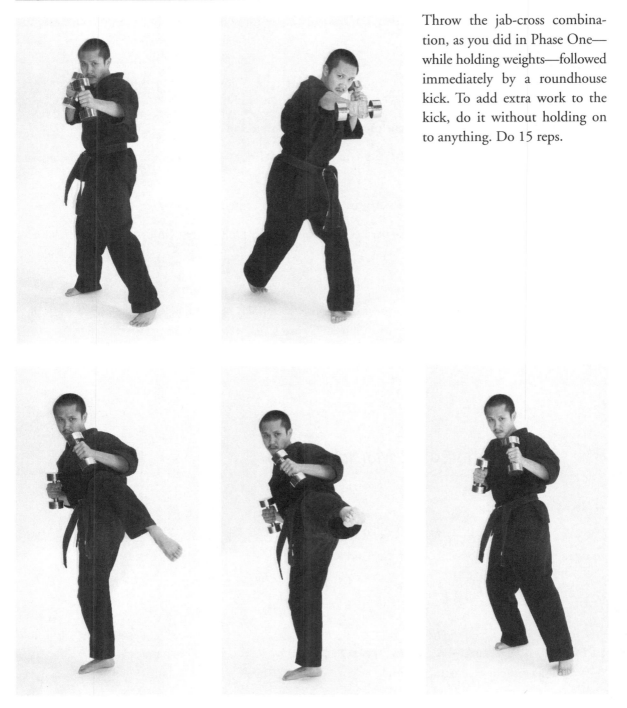

Throw the jab-cross combination, as you did in Phase One—while holding weights—followed immediately by a roundhouse kick. To add extra work to the kick, do it without holding on to anything. Do 15 reps.

C. 5-PUNCH, 1-KICK COMBINATION

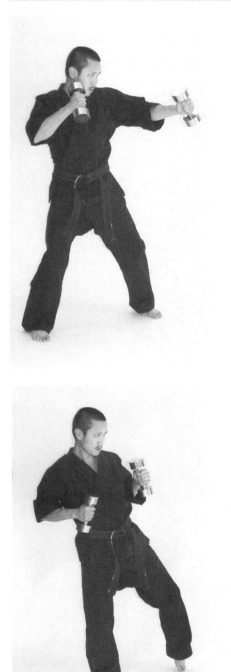

This combination consists of a jab-cross–roundhouse kick–jab-cross-hook. Do 20 reps while holding weights.

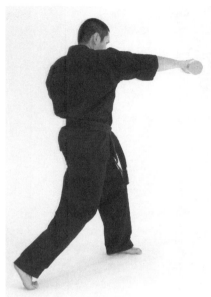

Perfect the Details: Focus on gracefulness, and not just sheer power. Try to make the combinations fluid and seamless. Allow the aggressive movements to relieve your stress. Stay quick, quick, quick! Float like a butterfly and sting like a bee!

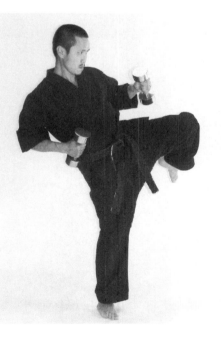

(continued on next page)

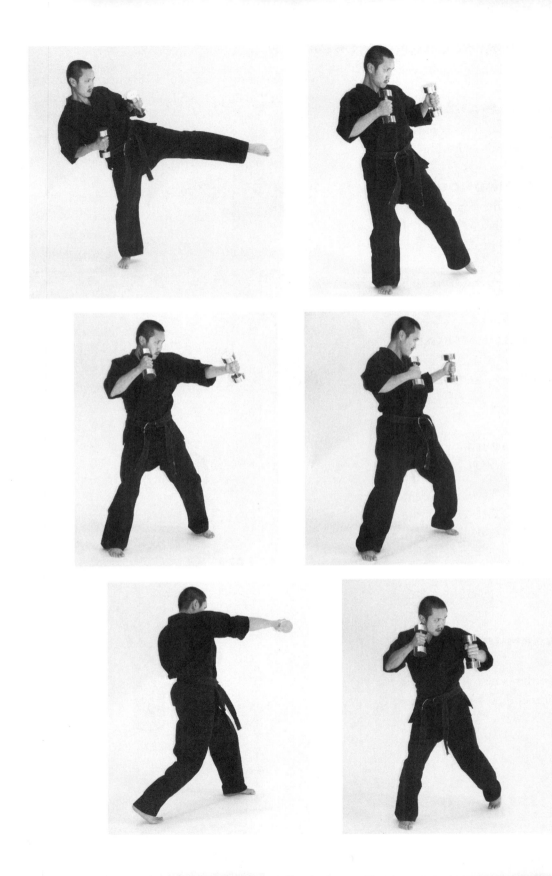

2. KICKS: At this level, you do 2 different kick combinations that will total a whopping 200 kicks. If this doesn't ignite your abs, nothing will.

A. SNAP-AND-ROUNDHOUSE-KICK COMBINATION: Do the snap-and-roundhouse combination as fast as you can. Alternate the snap and roundhouse. Be a blur! Go beyond the Breakthrough Moment. Do 25 of each kick, for a total of 50 kicks.

B. ROUNDHOUSE KICKS: Do 50 rapid-fire roundhouses, then switch sides and do 50 more with the other leg. After that, switch back to the first leg, and do 50 more. This totals 150 roundhouse kicks.

When you combine these roundhouses with the 50 snap-roundhouse combinations, you'll hit 200 kicks.

Perfect the Details: Think speed. Don't do the snap kick like a soccer kick, with a big windup— just flick it out. Once you set your femur, or thigh bone, in place, try not to move it.

3. THAI KNEE-ABS: Do this movement the same as before. But now ramp up your reps to 3 sets of 20 with each knee.

Perfect the Details: Be dynamic. Focus on your own power. Keep your mind in the movement, even though it's relatively simple. Keep your abs engaged.

COOLDOWN

Pamper yourself. Feel the sensual warmth in your muscles. Move them around. Bask in their heat. You're becoming a new you, aren't you?

Phase Three | Friday | *Core Interval Training Day*

WARM-UP

Do the same warm-up as in the 2 prior phases: 5 minutes of cardio, plus the 3-kick sequence. For a review of these kicks, see Phase One.

1. PUSH-UPS

Target: Your upper body and abs.

How-To: Same as in Phase Two, but this time you do more.

How Many: 20 reps or rep out: Do as many as you possibly can.

Perfect the Details: Focus on the supporting leg and arm, not the leg and arm that you're lifting. Keep your abs tight. Keep your weight evenly balanced. Keep breathing! Exhale as you push up.

2. STATIONARY CARDIO INTERVAL

Target: Your heart rate. In Phase Three, throttle it all the way up to 80 percent of your maximum rate.

How-To: Same as in Phase Two. Now, though, challenge yourself even more, by moving your arms in a way that is not natural for your body. For example, if you do jumping jacks, clasp your hands together, and swing them across the front of your body, in a diagonal line, from shoulder to hip.

How Long: 1 minute, 3 times, with short rests in between

Perfect the Details: Change your movement often. Do as many movements as your imagination will allow. Work harder than ever! There's no substitute for effort.

3. WIDE ROWS, WITH A SINGLE-LEG SQUAT

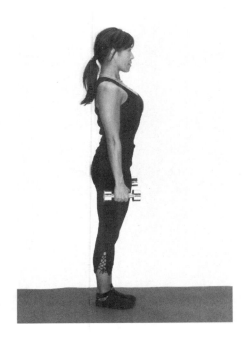

Target: Your upper back, shoulders, abdominals.

How-To: Same as in Phase Two, but add a squat. As you extend your arms toward the floor, slowly bend your supporting leg, to perform a single-leg squat. As you bend your elbows to row, slowly extend your supporting leg out of the squat, as pictured.

How Many: 8–10 with each leg

Perfect the Details: Focus on the specific muscles you're working. Visualize driving your weight through the floor. Don't arch your back. Keep your body flat and parallel to the floor.

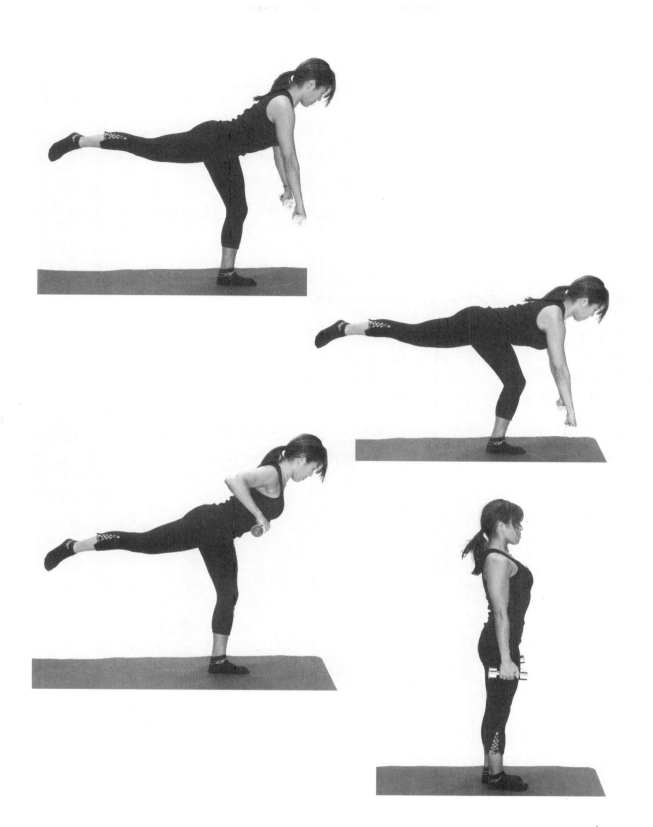

4. LATERAL-SHUFFLE CARDIO INTERVAL

Target: Your heart rate, and the muscles that control lateral movement. In this phase, crank your heart rate up to 80 percent of maximum.

How-To: Same as in Phase Two, but increase your distance and speed. Try to touch the markers you put on the floor, on each side of your shuffle.

How Long: 1 minute, 3 times, with short rests in between, for a total of 3 minutes

Perfect the Details: Pick your feet up. Keep your upper body steady and engaged. Visualize your heart getting stronger.

5. LUNGE-BALANCE WITH BICEP CURL AND SHOULDER PRESS

Target: Butt, abs, biceps, and shoulders.

How-To: Same as Phase Two. But as you step your feet together, instead of tapping your toe down, lift that knee and balance, as you perform the bicep curl, with your palms facing your shoulders. After that, as you press the dumbbells overhead, extend the bent knee straight out, as pictured.

How Many: 10–15 with each leg, alternating

Perfect the Details: Press your body's weight through your supporting hip and heel as you move. Live in your muscles. Don't arch your back as you press the weights overhead. If necessary, drop to a lower weight.

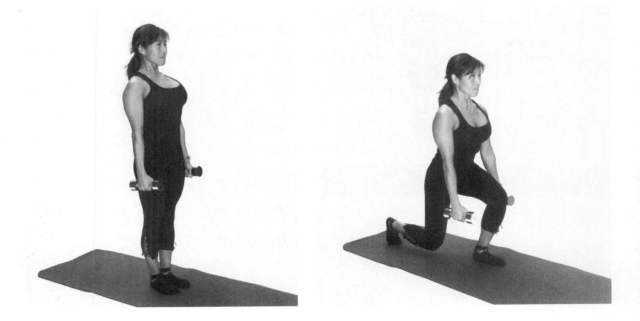

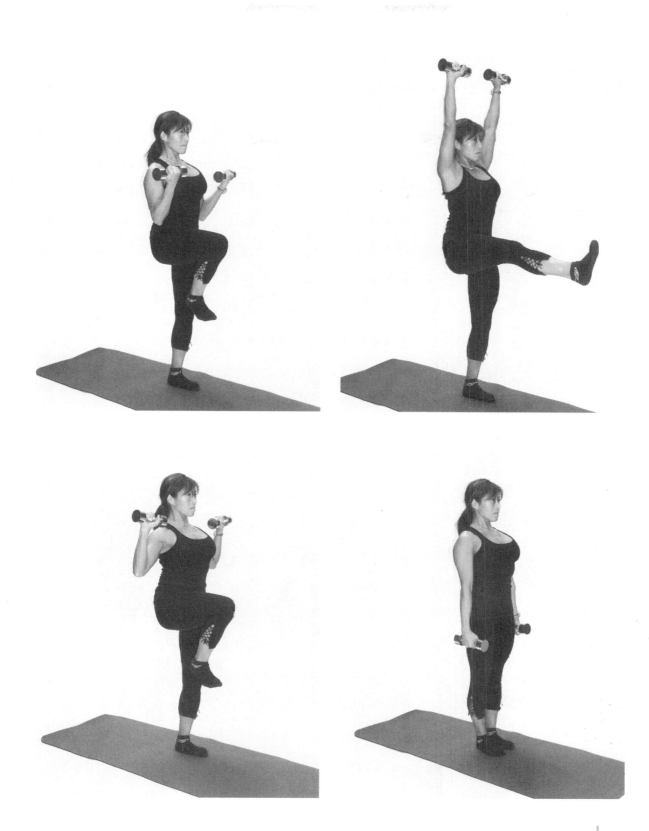

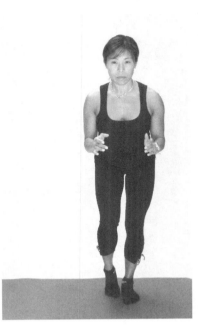

Target: Your heart rate: 80 percent of maximum—almost to the Breakthrough Moment. Also, your butt, core, and balance.

How-To: Same as in Phase Two. This time, though, completely balance on one leg as you land from the jump, as pictured. You can either lift the opposite knee, or bring the heel behind you.

How Many: 20–30 jumps on each side—for 40–60 total. Do this 3 times.

Perfect the Details: Pick up the pace—but don't sacrifice good form, balance, or control. Sink down into your supporting hip and heel as you land. Keep your head and chest up. Swing your arms from side to side, as if you were rollerblading.

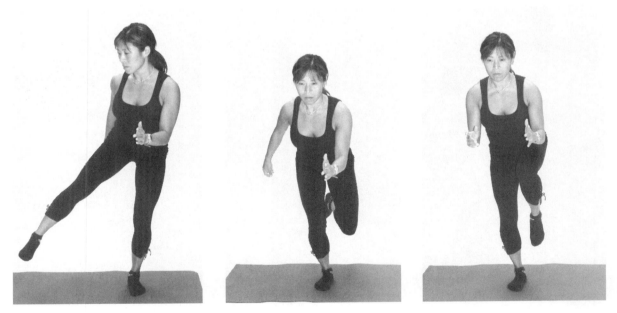

7. ABDOMINAL BICYCLE CRUNCHES, WITH TWISTS

Target: Your abs and obliques.

How-To: Same as in Phase Two, but now you add a new movement to your twist. As you rotate your upper body side to side, also create circular movements, as pictured. If you were standing upright, this would be similar to the movement of shoveling dirt and tossing it over your shoulder.

How Many: 20 pedals with each leg, for 40 total

Perfect the Details: Start the bicycle movement in your lower body first, then incorporate the circular movement in your upper body. Keep your legs as close together as possible. Keep your lower body centered, while your upper body rotates. Keep your torso grounded.

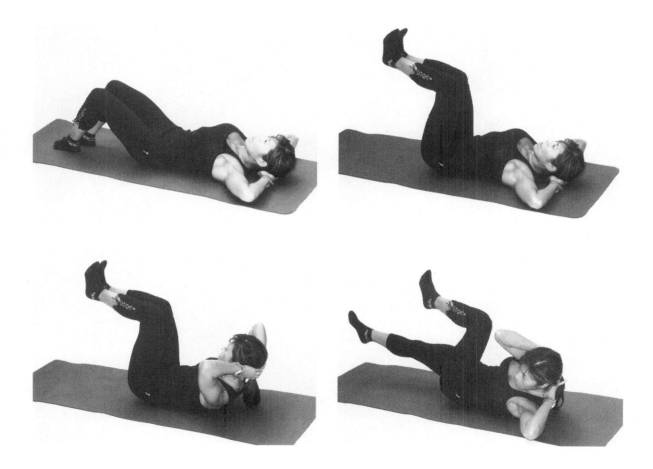

(continued on next page)

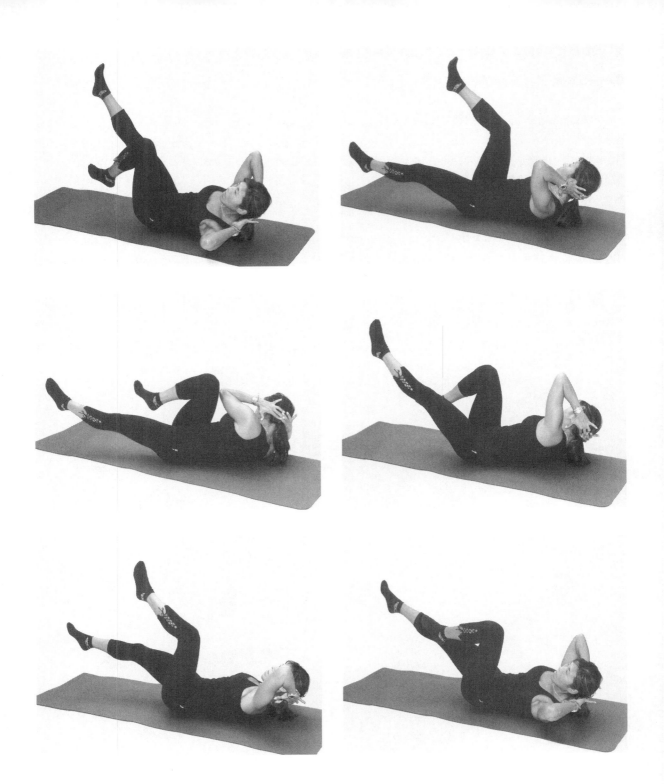

8. MOUNTAIN-CLIMBER COMBO CARDIO INTERVAL

Target: Your heart rate. Also, your abs, upper body, and core muscles.

How-To: Alternate the Phase One and Phase Two methods. Phase One: Bring your knees straight in. Phase Two: Bring your knees in to the opposite elbows.

How Many: Bring both knees straight in, then bring both knees in diagonally, 15 times. Then repeat it again, another 15 times.

Perfect the Details: Focus on your supporting leg, not the knee that bends. Keep your back as flat and stable as possible. Keep your shoulders and elbows in a straight line as you extend your chest forward.

COOLDOWN

Let your pumping heart slowly slide back to its normal range of heartbeat. Your heart is stronger now, so it will happen faster than it once did. You have changed!

Go into your last two weekends with vigor and zest. Do the physical activities that used to feel like work—a hike, or a bike ride. They're pure fun now, aren't they?

I'm proud of you.

Appendix D

The *One Body, One Life* Blueprint for Success

Getting Started

- Read, graze, and get familiar with the *One Body, One Life* concepts and material.
- Take the self-assessment survey and create your fitness mantra.
- Use the calorie calculator to establish your own daily calorie intake.
- Use the nutritional guidelines and sample menus to create your own daily menu plan for the week ahead. Then go shopping for these items—be prepared.

The First Two Weeks

- Use the techniques in Phase One to learn how to focus, allowing yourself to be fully present when performing the various tasks of this program.
- Eat according to the menu plan you have constructed, which should include three meals and three snacks each day.
- Perform the Phase One cleansing practice. Drink half your body weight in ounces of water daily and become aware of your breathing by daily practice of *kumbhaka* breathing and *ujjayi* breathing.
- Complete the Phase One workouts. Create your workout space and schedule your exercise time. Make your space sacred and your time the highest priority

The Next Two Weeks

- Talk to yourself when working out, and listen to your body and mind when you don't feel like exercising.
- Using the nutritional guidelines you learned in Phase One, implement a consistent eating routine that keeps you feeling continually satisfied.
- Take herbal supplements to help eliminate parasites. Perform the weekend cleanse for one day of weekends three and four.
- Complete the Phase Two workouts. Consider using aspirin to combat inflammation, should this arise as an issue. Always remember to consult a physician before practicing a medicinal regime.

The Final Two Weeks

- Focus on your posture, how you carry yourself, and your attitude. Learn to project yourself as the superstar you are.
- Study the fitness supplement list and begin a supplement regime that is outlined by this plan.
- Perform the weekend cleanse on both days of weekends five and six.
- Complete the Phase Three workouts. Work hard to find the Breakthrough Moment.

Beyond Week Six

- Integrate the four elements of fitness into one holistic plan. Mix and match your workouts, and find a routine that shapes itself around your new lifestyle.

About the Authors

Gregory Joujon-Roche is the founder of Holistic Fitness, a state-of-the-art fitness studio in California. He is the personal trainer to the stars, having worked with Brad Pitt for the film *Troy*, Tobey Maguire for his superhero physique in *Spider-Man*, and Demi Moore for her preparation for the film *G.I. Jane*—among many others. Since its inception in 1994, Holistic Fitness has grown to include a team of the finest doctors, cooks, masseuses, yoga instructors, martial artists, and fitness experts available. Joujon-Roche lives in California.

Cameron Stauth has written twenty-two books, including several national and international bestsellers. His books have been published in twelve languages, and have had an impact upon health protocols and medical practice in America and abroad. He has written articles for publications such as *The New York Times Magazine*, *Esquire*, and *Prevention*. *The New York Times* has called him "a tireless reporter and a talented and graceful writer." Among his books are *The Franchise*, *The New Approach to Cancer*, *What Happy People Know*, and *Brain Longevity*.

Index